Changes in
Health and Medicine
c. 1345 to the present day

Colin P. F. Hughes

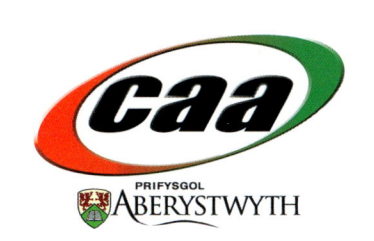

Changes in Health and Medicine, c. 1345 to the present day

© Aberystwyth University, 2013

Published by CAA, Aberystwyth University, Gogerddan Mansion, Aberystwyth, Ceredigion, SY23 3EB (www.aber.ac.uk/caa)
Sponsored by the Welsh Government

ISBN: 978-1-84521-525-5

These materials are subject to copyright and may not be reproduced or published in any form without the permission of the copyright holder. All rights reserved.

Editor: Lynwen Rees Jones
Designer: Richard Huw Pritchard
Source research and copyright clearing: Gwenda Lloyd Wallace
Printed by: Cambrian Printers

The publisher would like to thank:
The Monitoring Panel: Anne Carroll, Jami Davies, Sarah Horton, Anwen Môn Jones, Alun Millington and Deiniol Williams, for their valuable guidance.

Professor Phillipp Schofield, Department of History and Welsh History, Aberystwyth University, for his valuable comments on the text.

Thank you to the following for kind permission to reproduce illustrations:

Michal Pober, Founder and Director of the former Alchemy Museum in Kutná Hora: p. 2(l)

Wellcome Library, London: pp. 2(r), 3(l), 7, 14, 16, 17, 22, 23, 26, 32, 37, 39, 40, 41, 42, 43(r), 44, 45(l), 46, 51, 52, 53, 56, 58, 62, 64, 65, 71, 78(b,l), 91

Science & Society Picture Library: pp. 3(r), 5(l), 8, 10, 11(t,r), 27(b,l), 43(l), 57, 106(t)

Topfoto: pp. 5(r), 27(t,l), 29(r), 30, 34, 49, 54, 68, 81, 94(l), 105(t)

Royal Collection Trust / © Her Majesty Queen Elizabeth II 2013: p. 12

Getty Images: pp. 24, 38, 96, 97

Science Photo Library: pp. 27(b,r), 28, 29(l), 50(r), 69(t), 72, 98(r), 110

Oxford University Press: Catrin Stevens, *Discovering Welsh History: Book 2: Wales in the Middle Ages* (Oxford: Oxford University Press, 1992), pp. 46-7: p. 36

Mary Evans Picture Library: pp. 45(r), 94(r), 113

© The Hunterian Museum at the Royal College of Surgeons: p. 50(l)

Blond McIndoe Research Foundation: p. 67

The estate of A. L. Evans: p. 78(t)

City & County of Swansea: Swansea Museums Collection: p. 86(l)

© Crown Copyright: Royal Commission on the Ancient and Historical Monuments of Wales: p. 86(r)

© National Museum of Wales: p. 88(l)

© Copyright Jeremy Lowe: pp. 88(r), 89

Hodder Education: Ben Walsh, *GCSE British Social & Economic History*, 'History in Focus' (London: Hodder Murray, 1997), p. 197: p. 92(r)

© Heritage Images: pp. 95, 98(l)

National Library of Wales: p. 99

Fflur Aneira Davies: p. 103

Elen Jones: p. 104

© Solo Syndication/National Library of Wales: Leslie Gilbert Illingworth, 'Here's to the brave new world!', *Daily Mail*, 2 December 1942: p. 105(b)

© Mirrorpix/British Cartoon Archive, University of Kent, www.cartoons.ac.uk: Vicky (Victor Weisz), 'Here he comes, boys!', *Daily Mirror*, 7 August 1945: p. 106(b)

© Express Newspapers/British Cartoon Archive, University of Kent, www.cartoons.ac.uk: Ronald Carl Giles, 'Dentist says if there are any more … ', *Daily Express*, 22 December 1949: p. 107

Thank you to the following for kind permission to reproduce extracts:

Oxford University Press: Irvine Loudon (ed.), *Western Medicine: An Illustrated History* (Oxford: Oxford University Press, 1997): pp. 12 (p. 78), 13 (p. 77), 22 (p. 102-3), 26 (p. 109), 62 (p. 118), 69 (p. 184)

Norman Publishing: Andreas Vesalius, *De Humani Corporis Fabrica Libri Septem*, trans. by William Frank Richardson, in collaboration with John Burd Carman: *On the Fabric of the Human Body, Book 1: The Bones and Cartilages* (San Francisco: Norman Publishing, 1998), p. 107: p. 15

Hodder Education: © Ian Dawson and Ian Coulson 1996, *Medicine and Health through Time: an SHP development study*, 'Discovering the Past for GCSE' (London: John Murray, 1996): pp. 15 (p. 84), 17 (p. 86), 18(r) (p. 88), 46 (p. 119), 109 (p. 169)

Donaldson IML (2004). 'Ambroise Paré's account in the Oeuvres of 1575 of new methods of treating gunshot wounds and burns.' JLL Bulletin: *Commentaries on the history of treatment evaluation* (www.jameslindlibrary.org): p. 16

Yale J Biol Med. 2002 Jan-Feb; 75(1): 59–62, Translated by Tina Dasgupta, Yale Journal of Biology and Medicine Original Contributions Editor: p. 25

Anova Book Group: Linda Pollock (ed.), *With Faith and Physic: The Life of a Tudor Gentlewoman, Lady Grace Mildmay, 1552-1620* (London: Collins & Brown, 1993): p. 37 (p. 137), 39 (p. 110), 40 (p. 138)

The Women's Library, London Metropolitan University (WL Vault C. Bentinck, 910.40924 WOR): John Cleland (ed.), *Letters of the Right Honourable Lady Montagu. Written during her travels in Europe, Asia and Africa, Vollume II*, 1st edition 1763, pp. 59-62. p. 43

Eaglemoss Publications Ltd: William Armstrong, 'Under the Surgeon's knife', *History Makers: The Magazine that brings History to Life* (London: Marshall Cavendish, Sidgwick & Jackson, 30 January 1970), pp. 466-9: pp. 52, 55

With thanks to the Royal College of Surgeons Edinburgh for their assistance: p. 54(r)

Peter Mantin and Richard Pulley: Peter Mantin and Richard Pulley, *Medicine Through the Ages* (Cheltenham: Stanley Thornes (Publishers) Ltd, 1997): pp. 56 (p. 41), 64 (p. 110)

The Royal College of Surgeons of England: Minutes of Council. 1911-1913, p. 132. Tribute presented at the Ordinary Council Meeting, 14 March, 1912 (London: The Royal College of Surgeons of England, 1913): p. 57

John Rowlands: p. 58

Oxford Brookes University Medical Sciences Video Archive: p. 65(r)

Medical Research Council: Letter from H.W. Florey to E. Mellanby, 6 September 1939: Medical Research Council file FD1/3334, kept at The National Archives: p. 65(l)

Curtis Brown Group Ltd, London on behalf of The Estate of André Maurois 1959. Copyright © André Maurois: André Maurois, *The Life of Alexander Fleming: Discoverer of Penicillin* (New York: E.P. Dutton & Co, Inc., 1959), pp. 179-180: p. 66

With thanks to the Blond McIndoe Research Foundation for their assistance: pp. 66-67

Bishop Peter Price, Diocese of Bath & Wells/Somerset Record Society: taken from *The register of Thomas Bekynton, Bishop of Bath and Wells, 1443-1465*, edited by Sir H.C. Maxwell-Lyte and M.C.B. Dawes (Somerset Record Society, vols 49-50, 1934-35): p. 78(c,r)

© Cambridge University Press: Miri Rubin, *Charity and Community in Medieval Cambridge* (Cambridge: Cambridge University Press, 1987), pp. 300-301: p. 78(b,r)

© Cambridge University Press: Vanessa Harding, *The Dead and the Living in Paris and London* (Cambridge: Cambridge University Press, 2002), pp. 19-21, 116: p. 79

Manchester University Press: Rosemary Horrox, *The Black Death* (Manchester: Manchester University Press, 1994), p. 63: p. 80

Dafydd Johnston: Dafydd Johnston (ed. and trans.), *Galar y Beirdd/Poet's Grief* (Cardiff: Tafol, 1993), pp. 51, 53: p. 80

Oxford University Press: Henry Mayhew, *London Labour and the London Poor: A Selected Edition,* ed. Robert Douglas-Fairhurst (Oxford: Oxford University Press, 2012), p. 435: p. 87

With thanks to the National Library of Wales for their assistance (Cwrtmawr MS. 393): p. 87(b,r)

With thanks to the National Library of Wales: G. Penrhyn Jones, 'Cholera in Wales', *The National Library of Wales Journal,* Vol. 10, No. 3, Summer 1958, pp. 287, 295: p. 89(b), 90(c and b)

With thanks to Lincolnshire Archives for their assistance: p. 92

University College London Library Services: Special Collections, Chadwick Papers 2181/1: p. 93

Courtesy of St Bartholomew's Hospital Archives. Volume ref. SBHB/HA/1/9 f.63 verso (minutes of the board of governors): p. 97

Eric Birbeck MVO: Eric Birbeck, 'The Royal Hospital Haslar: from Lind to the 21st century', 2011: p. 97

The British Library: Letter from Florence Nightingale to her father, 22 February 1854: MS 45790 f. 157: p. 97

Roger Turvey: Roger Turvey, *Wales and Britain 1906-1951* (London: Hodder & Stoughton Educational, a division of Hodder Headline Plc, 1997), p. 152: p. 106

Quartet Books: Aneurin Bevan, *In Place of Fear* (London: Quartet Books, 1990), pp. 99-101: p. 106

© Solo Syndication: 'The watch on your life', John Hall, *Daily Mail*, 3 July 1948, p. 2: p. 107

Office for National Statistics: p. 109

Copyright Guardian News & Media Ltd 2011: p. 109

BBC News at bbc.co.uk/news: p. 110

The publisher's diligent attempts at tracing the copyright holders of the following sources have been unsuccessful. They would be pleased to hear from the copyright holders in order to make suitable arrangements.

Dorothy Fisk, *Doctor Jenner of Berkeley* (London: William Heinemann Ltd, 1959), pp. 117-8: p. 44

Martha Marquardt, *Paul Ehrlich* (New York: Henry Schuman, 1951), pp. 168-9, 173: p. 62

George Holmes: *The Later Middle Ages, 1272-1485* (Edinburgh: Thomas Nelson and Sons, 1962), p. 136: p. 82

A Welsh medium version of this publication is also available: *Newidiadau ym maes Iechyd a Meddygaeth tua 1345 hyd heddiw*

Contents

Issue 1: Developments in medical knowledge

01	Chapter 1	What were the main medical ideas common in Wales and England in the late Middle Ages?
09	Chapter 2	What were the main developments in medical knowledge in the sixteenth and seventeenth centuries?
21	Chapter 3	How much progress has been made in medical knowledge from the nineteenth century to today?

Issue 2: Changes in the prevention and treatment of diseases

35	Chapter 4	How did methods of treating disease in Wales and England change from the late Middle Ages to the eighteenth century?
49	Chapter 5	What were the main advances made in surgical methods in Britain in the nineteenth century?
61	Chapter 6	What have been the main turning points in the prevention and treatment of disease from the twentieth century to today?

Issue 3: Developments in public health and patient care in Wales and England

77	Chapter 7	How were the sick cared for in Wales and England from the late Middle Ages to the eighteenth century?
85	Chapter 8	What were the main advances in public health and patient care in Wales and England in the nineteenth century?
103	Chapter 9	How has health care in Wales and England improved from the twentieth century to today?
115		Glossary

CHAPTER 1

WHAT WERE THE MAIN MEDICAL IDEAS COMMON IN WALES AND ENGLAND IN THE LATE MIDDLE AGES?

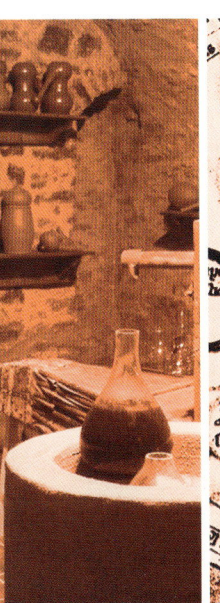

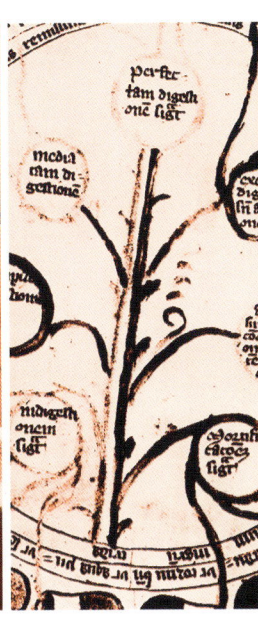

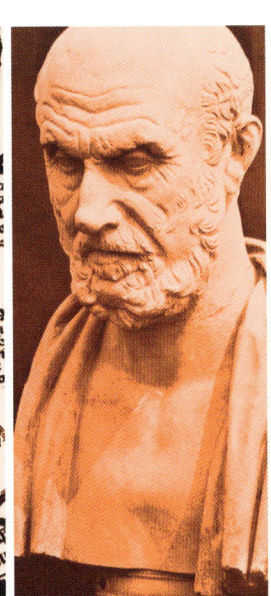

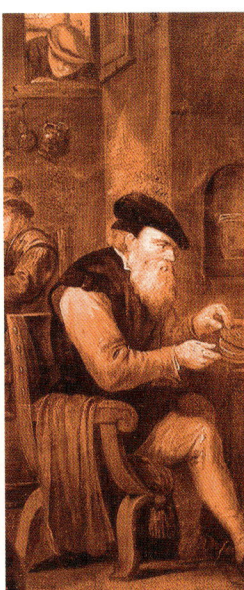

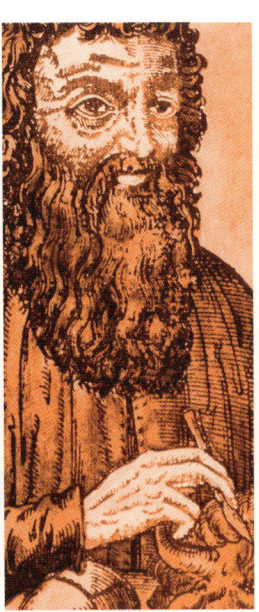

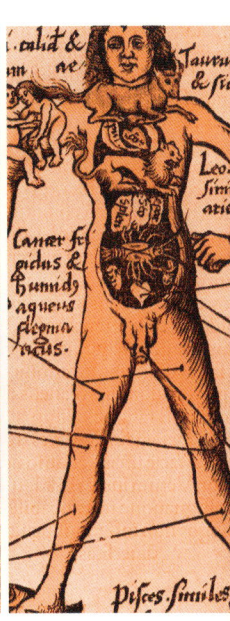

THE IDEA OF ALCHEMY

People have always wanted to live longer and healthier lives. Over the centuries, this has resulted in many new ideas and many developments in medical knowledge and understanding. One popular idea in the Middle Ages, which had been in existence since ancient times, was **alchemy**. Alchemists believed that there was a strong link between people's lives and the cosmos, or universe. The two main aims of alchemy were to create the legendary 'philosopher's stone', which could turn **base metals** into gold or silver, and to produce the 'elixir of life', a potion that could make a person immortal or forever young.

Alchemy had originated in the ancient civilisations of China, India and Greece but had become unpopular because of its association with magic and superstition. It eventually re-emerged in ancient Egypt, where it came to be regarded as a subject worthy of serious study. From there, it moved to Europe in the late Middle Ages when ancient writings were translated into Latin, the common written language of the time, and finally to Britain.

Alchemy in the Middle Ages was a mixture of science, philosophy and mysticism. One of the first Englishmen to study the subject was Roger Bacon (1214-92). After studying at Oxford and the University of Paris, he became interested in philosophy, magic and alchemy.

The search for drugs and potions

At the heart of medieval alchemy was the idea that all matter was composed of four elements: earth, air, fire and water. Each of these elements was believed to have different qualities that could be observed from the natural world during the different seasons:

- Earth was cold and dry in autumn;
- Air was hot and moist in spring;
- Fire was hot and dry in summer;
- Water was cold and moist in winter.

With the right combination of these elements, alchemists believed that any substance on earth could be created.

Although alchemists did not succeed in finding the philosopher's stone, in the process they did develop new equipment and new technology for extracting chemicals, refining liquids and mixing potions, which became useful in preparing herbal remedies.

SOURCE 1

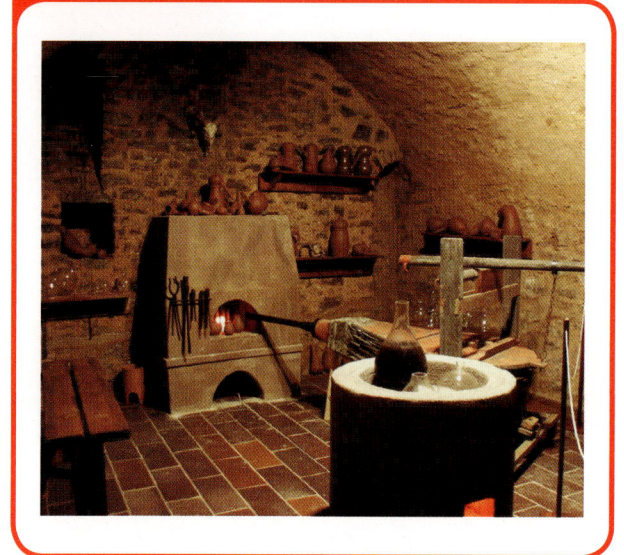

A reconstruction of a medieval alchemist's laboratory showing some of the equipment used

Alchemists continued their searches throughout the late Middle Ages for the elusive 'elixir of life', believing that it could be a cure for all diseases. Despite opposition to some of their ideas, they used their developing science to make advances in medicine:
- Medieval alchemists produced hydrochloric acid, nitric acid, potash and sodium carbonate;
- Alchemists were able to identify the elements arsenic, antimony and bismuth (which were to be used in medicines);
- Through their experiments, medieval alchemists invented and developed laboratory equipment that is, in modified form, still used today;
- The practice of alchemy laid the foundation for the development of chemistry as a scientific discipline.

Without these achievements, modern **pharmacology**, so important in treating today's illnesses, might not have been possible.

The idea of alchemy continued to fascinate enquiring minds until well into the sixteenth and seventeenth centuries. Dr John Dee (1527-1608) was an adviser to Queen Elizabeth I. He was born in London but his father was from Radnorshire (in the modern-day county of Powys) and originally spelled his surname 'Du' (black). John Dee was multi-talented and wrote books on alchemy and **astrology**, as well as on various other subjects. He even claimed to have found a quantity of the elixir of life in the ruins of Glastonbury Abbey. His eldest son, Arthur, was also an alchemist.

SOURCE 2

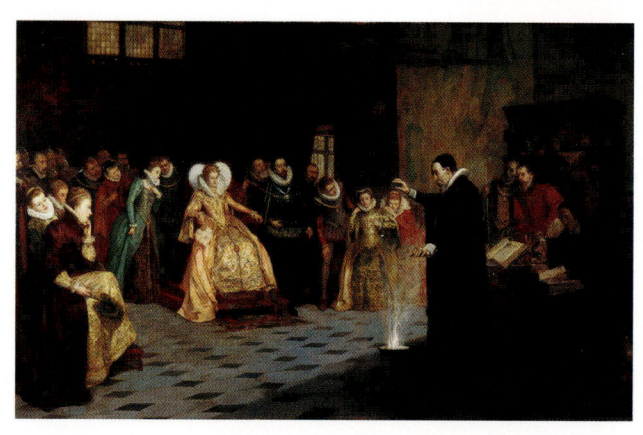

Dr John Dee, Elizabethan alchemist and astrologer demonstrating an experiment to Elizabeth I

TASKS

1. What is alchemy? Describe the achievements of the alchemists.
2. What does Source 1 tell you about alchemists?

OTHER COMMON IDEAS

If someone wanted to be a doctor in the Middle Ages, they had to train at a university medical school. A trained doctor was called a 'physician' – from the word 'physic' meaning healing. The physician was trained to use various methods to treat a patient, including the use of a urine chart.

SOURCE 3

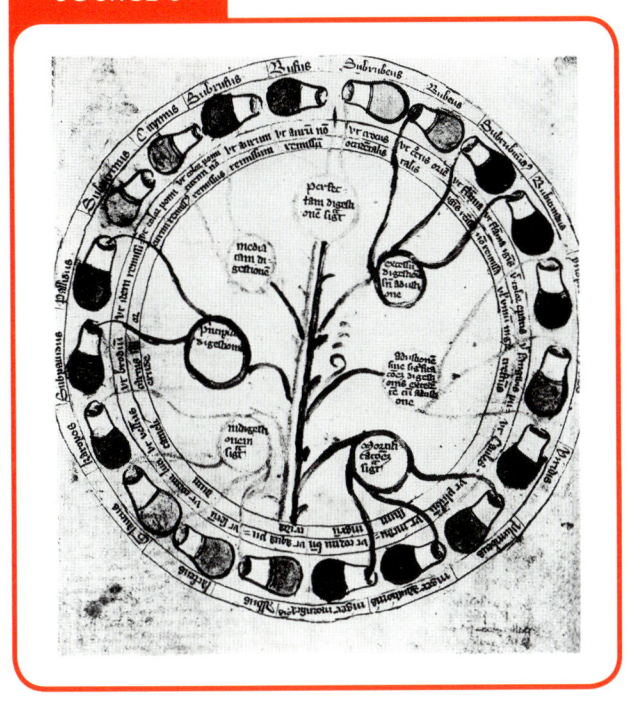

A urine chart

The urine chart showed different colours or shades of urine. A doctor could check a patient's urine sample against the chart and make a diagnosis on their health.

However, the medieval doctor also had other ideas and methods for treating patients, some of which were to do with superstition.

'Zodiac man' charts and the influence of astrology

Most of the important medical ideas in the Middle Ages were based on astrology. Trained doctors studied star charts, as they believed that the movement of the planets affected people's health. They studied the influence of the stars on the human body and carefully charted the results. Medieval doctors carried a *vademecum*, which was a pocket reference book containing the signs of the zodiac and 'zodiac man' charts. They would consult the chart and the position of the stars before making a diagnosis.

SOURCE 4

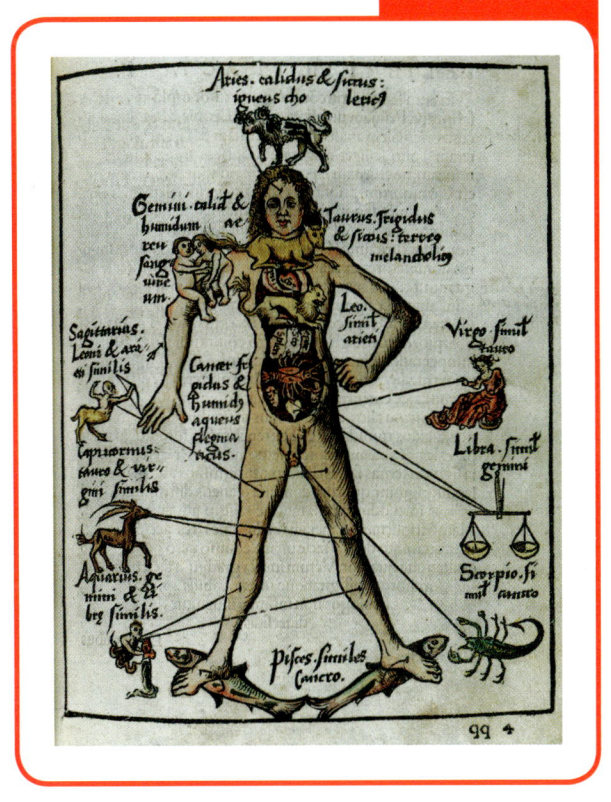

A zodiac man chart

Each sign of the zodiac, or star sign, was associated with different parts of the body and trained doctors would avoid operating on that part when certain stars were in the sky. For example, the chart above shows zodiac man with the Aries ram balanced on his head, so operations on the head were to be avoided when Aries was in the sky. Doctors believed that Libra, the sign of the balance, or scales, ruled the kidneys. They would therefore avoid operating on the kidneys when Libra was in the sky. The kidneys are the organs that maintain the balance of fluids (humours) in the body. The idea of the balance of the humours was an essential one in medieval times, as we shall see later.

The following list relates to the zodiac man chart above. Follow the star signs in a clockwise direction from the Aries ram on the zodiac man's head to see the advice given to medieval physicians.

3

Aries	Avoid incisions in the head and face and cut no vein on the head.
Taurus	Avoid incisions in the neck and throat and cut no veins there.
Leo	Avoid incisions of the nerves and the sides and do not cut the back.
Virgo	Avoid opening a wound in the belly and in internal parts.
Libra	Avoid opening wounds in the umbilicus and parts of the belly.
Scorpio	Avoid cutting the testicles and anus.
Pisces	(Zodiac man is standing on Pisces – the fish.) Avoid cutting the feet.
Aquarius	Avoid cutting the legs and places as far as the heels.
Capricorn	Avoid cutting the knees or the veins and sinews in these places.
Cancer	Avoid incisions in the breast and sides, stomach and lungs.
Sagittarius	Avoid incisions in the thighs and fingers and do not cut blemishes or growths.
Gemini	Avoid incisions in the shoulders and arms or hands and cut no vein.

Some medieval astrologers were thought to be magicians, but others were highly respected scholars. Some of the ideas above may seem superstitious today, but people firmly believed in them at the time. Indeed, people believed so strongly in these ideas that, even beyond the Middle Ages and into the sixteenth century, doctors across Europe were required by law to calculate the position of the moon before carrying out medical procedures, such as surgery or bleeding.

The theory of the four humours

The theory of the four humours dominated medical ideas for almost two thousand years. It was developed by ancient Greek and Roman doctors and remained popular until the mid nineteenth century.

According to the theory, the body contained four important liquids called humours, which were related to the four seasons:
- Blood (Spring);
- Yellow bile (Summer);
- Black bile (Autumn);
- Phlegm (Winter).

If the humours stayed in balance, then the person remained healthy. If the humours became unbalanced (if there was too much of one humour and not enough of another) then illness occurred.

Doctors in ancient Greece had tried to understand what caused illness by carefully observing people who were unwell. When someone was ill, they observed that a liquid would usually be discharged from the body, such as phlegm from the nose or vomit from the stomach. They believed that this liquid, or humour, was the cause of the illness and that it was removed from the body because there was too much of it – the humours were out of balance.

The theory of the four humours grew directly from the theory of the four elements. We have already seen that medieval alchemy was based on the idea that all matter was composed of four elements: earth, air, fire and water.

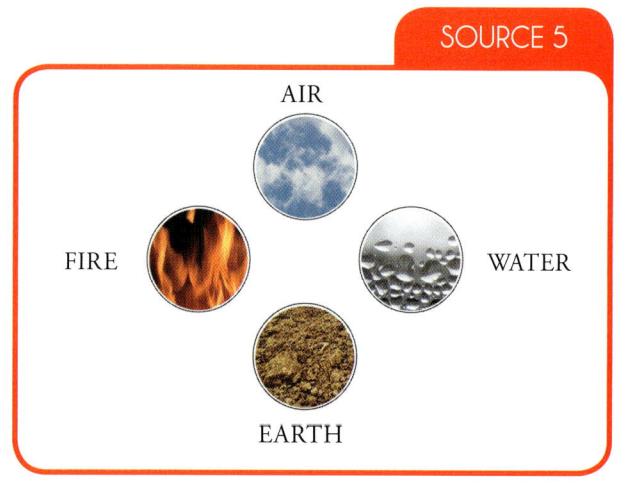

SOURCE 5

The four elements

The ancient Greeks had linked the four seasons with the four elements and their different qualities.

SOURCE 6

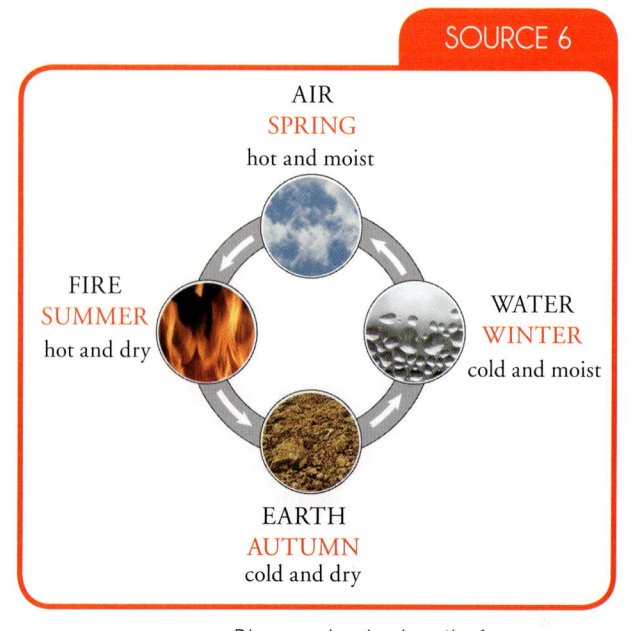

Diagram showing how the four seasons were linked to the four elements

Greek doctors had observed that people were often ill in winter with sneezing and runny noses. They believed that these people had too much phlegm, the humour most like water, which was cold and moist, just like the winter season. They also believed that the humours were the cause of illness and that it was important, therefore, to keep the patient's body in balance. They did this by removing excess fluid:
- Excess blood was removed by bleeding into a bowl or by using a leech;
- Excess bile could be removed with a **purgative** like mustard water to make the patient vomit.

TASKS

1. What does Source 3 show you about medical ideas in the Middle Ages?
2. Why was a *vademecum* important for medieval doctors?
3. Describe the theory of the four humours.

Continuity of ideas

In the Middle Ages the medical ideas of Hippocrates and Galen were still followed. These men had helped to develop the theory of the four humours as well as other ideas in the field of medicine.

Hippocrates

SOURCE 7

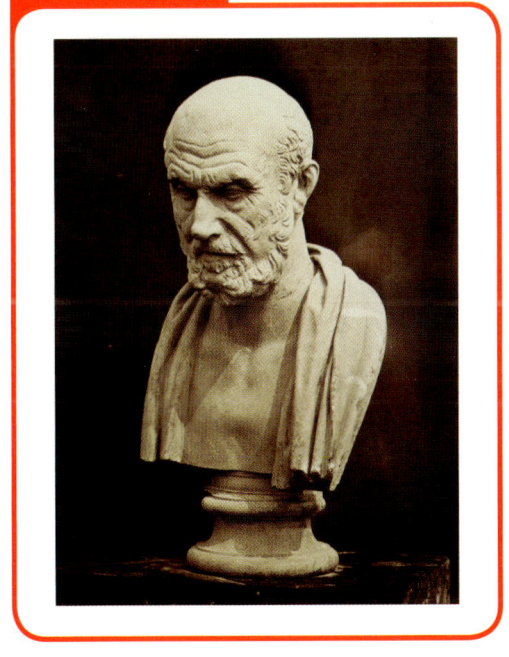

Hippocrates of Kos

Hippocrates was a Greek doctor who taught medicine in the fourth century BC. He wrote a number of medical books, advising doctors how to treat their patients. He taught that, in order to cure a patient, doctors should observe and record carefully the symptoms and developments of diseases. This method is still used today and is called **clinical observation**.

Hippocrates developed the theory of the four humours to explain the causes of disease and he also encouraged people to look for natural treatments for illnesses, rather than praying to the gods for help. Because of his ideas, Hippocrates has been called 'The Father of Modern Medicine'.

Galen

SOURCE 8

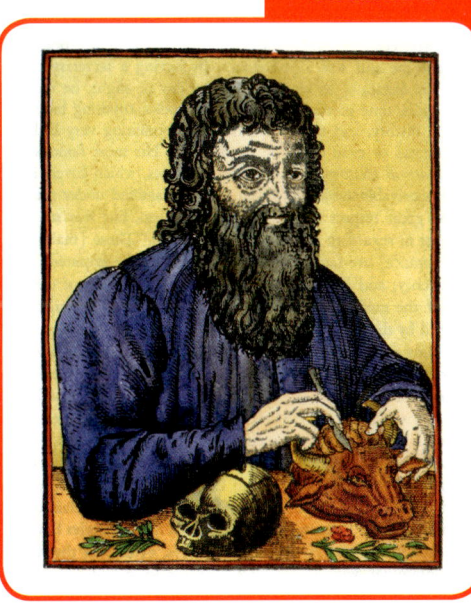

Galen – Aelius Galenus or Claudius Galenus

Galen was born in Greece in about 130 AD. He wrote several books on medicine. He learned a lot about the anatomy of the human body by treating the wounds of gladiators. Human dissection was forbidden at that time, so this was a very useful way for Galen to increase his knowledge of the structure of the human body. Galen emphasised the importance of Hippocrates' methods of observation and recording. Like

Hippocrates, he also believed in the theory of the four humours, but he had different ideas about restoring the balance of the humours.

There are three main reasons why these medical ideas lasted for such a long time. Firstly people believed in traditional methods of dealing with illness; secondly there were limited numbers of books to spread new ideas and finally communication across the developed world was slow and often interrupted by warfare.

The end of the Middle Ages

There was little improvement in doctors' understanding of illness and disease throughout the Middle Ages. In general, doctors continued to follow the ideas of the ancient writers and the theory of the four humours.

However, there were some doctors who had different ideas about illness. Their most powerful idea was that God and the Devil influenced health. They believed that epidemics like the Black Death were punishments from God for people's sins. However, they also believed that God could cure people. Astrology continued to be important, but doctors began to realise that there was a link between dirt and disease, although they did not know yet what the link was.

We now know that the ideas of some ancient medical writers contained errors. However, there seemed to be little desire to change or to challenge the old ideas. It was not until the **Renaissance** began in the late fifteenth and early sixteenth centuries that any great advances in medical knowledge were to be made.

TASKS

1. Explain why doctors believed in the ancient ideas on medicine for so long.
2. Describe some ideas on medical knowledge that were different from the theory of the four humours.
3. What eventually changed the ancient medical ideas from about 1500?

Examination practice

This section provides guidance on how to answer Question 1(a), 2(a) and 3(a) from Unit 3. It is a source comprehension question, which is worth 2 marks. The source could be a photograph, a cartoon, a map, a graph or a written account.

Question 1(a), 2(a), 3(a) – comprehension of a source

What does Source A show you about alchemists? [2 marks]

SOURCE A

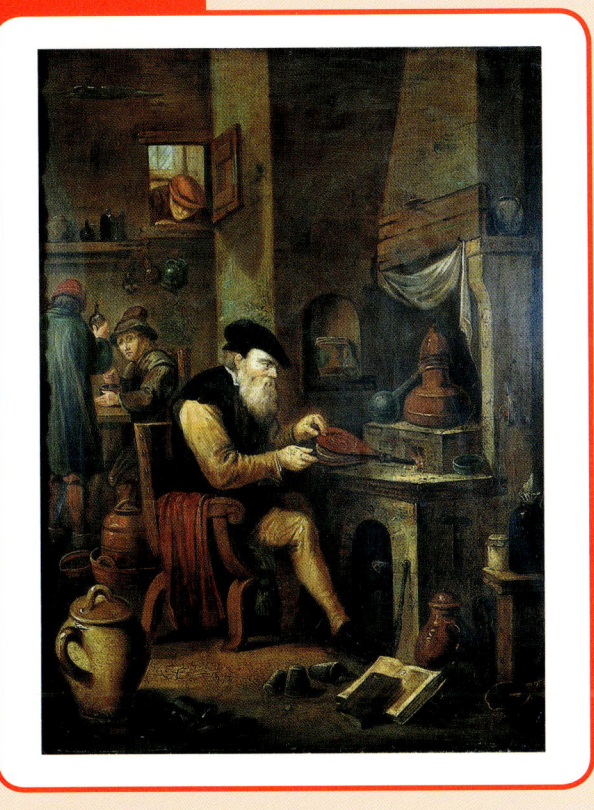

An alchemist at work in his laboratory

Tips on how to answer

- This is an inference question involving the comprehension of a visual source.
- You are asked to **pick out relevant information** from the source.
- You must also **make use of the statement written below the source**, which is intended to provide you with additional information.
- You must **only comment on the information that you can extract** from the source and what is written immediately below it. **Do not** bring in additional factual knowledge, as this will not score you marks.
- To obtain maximum marks you will need to pick out at least **two relevant points**.

Candidate response

Source A shows an alchemist working in a laboratory. He seems to be working on an experiment, using a bellows and some apparatus. He is using a book that is lying open at his feet. He has other people working with him at a table in the background of his dark laboratory.

Examiner's comment

The candidate has picked valid points from both the picture and the statement written below it. There is an understanding about the alchemist and the work that he does. This is a developed answer worthy of maximum (2) marks.

Now you have a go

What does Source B show you about a 'zodiac man' chart?

[2 marks]

SOURCE B

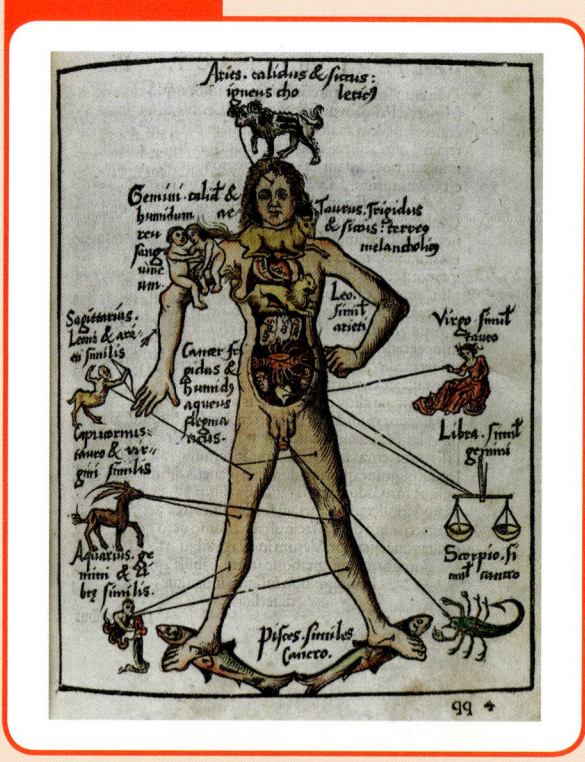

A zodiac man chart showing star signs linked to different parts of the human body

CHAPTER 2

WHAT WERE THE MAIN DEVELOPMENTS IN MEDICAL KNOWLEDGE IN THE SIXTEENTH AND SEVENTEENTH CENTURIES?

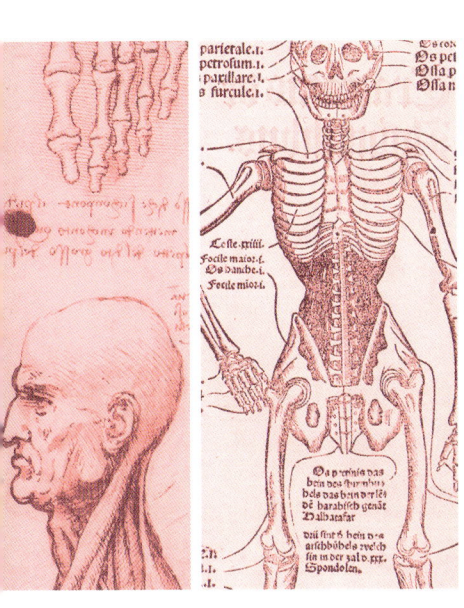

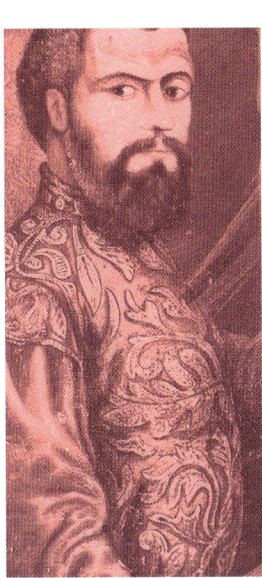

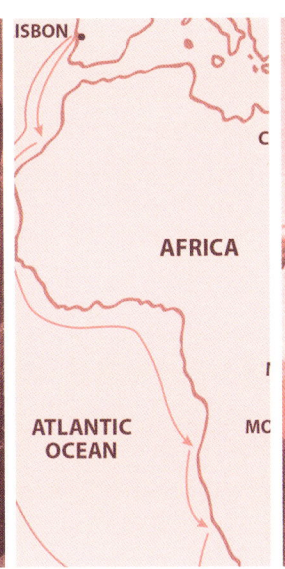

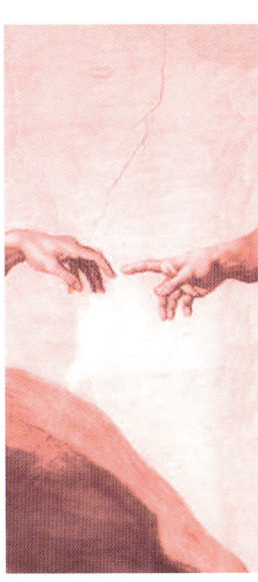

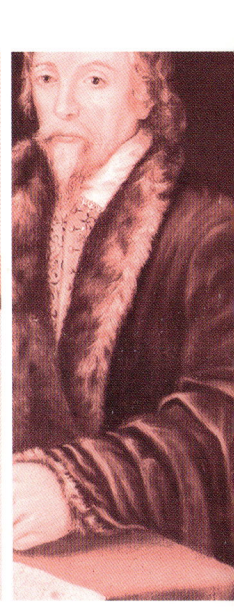

THE IMPACT OF THE RENAISSANCE

The influence of Renaissance ideas

Developments in medical knowledge had been very slow in the late Middle Ages, as physicians continued to follow ideas that had been in existence for over a thousand years. There had been a reluctance to change or to challenge the old ideas until, during the 15th century, there was a new movement called the **Renaissance**.

By the sixteenth century ideas were changing. The Renaissance, or 'rebirth', had influenced many aspects of learning across Europe, including literature, philosophy, politics, science and religion. New styles of art, music and architecture were also developed. After Constantinople fell to the Ottoman Turks in the mid fifteenth century, many of the Greek scholars that lived there fled to Italy, bringing with them ancient texts. This led to a renewed interest in the work of the ancient Europeans, particularly in Italy where scholars were already aware of the many achievements of the ancient Romans. Alchemists became interested in experimenting for themselves rather than accepting traditional ideas without question, and the more scientific approach of gathering evidence through research became popular.

Due to this change in attitude during the Renaissance period, rapid progress was made in medical knowledge and understanding, as well as in many other areas of learning.

The printing press

Another factor that increased the spread of learning during the Renaissance was the invention of the printing press.

SOURCE 1

the invention and spread of the printing press are widely regarded as among the most influential events in the second millennium [AD,] revolutionizing the way people conceive [understand] and describe the world they live in, and ushering [bringing] in the period of modernity.

From an Internet website

In the mid fifteenth century Johannes Gutenberg (c.1398-1468), a German blacksmith, goldsmith and inventor, developed a complete mechanical printing system, which led to the first ever mass production of books. A single printing press could print 3,600 pages in one day. This was a huge improvement on the 40 hand-printed pages by the previous system. Medical books from older civilisations were now printed and doctors began to study them in detail and challenge some long-held traditional ideas.

From Gutenberg's hometown in Germany, printing quickly spread to over 200 cities in many European countries. William Caxton (c.1422-92) was the first person to introduce a printing press to Britain and he was the first English person to sell printed books. Caxton set up a printing press at Westminster in London in 1476 and most of his work was printed in the English language, rather than the traditional Latin.

The invention of the printing press allowed the spread of professional medical ideas. After 1500, medical knowledge that had previously been restricted to professional physicians was made available to many more people.

Some wealthy women were able to take advantage of this new printing technology and they began to create their own medical libraries and private recipe collections. The Elizabethan gentlewoman Lady Grace Mildmay, for example, received some education in herbal medicine, as well as in minor surgery. She supplemented this with knowledge that she acquired from reading various medical books and developed an impressive collection of remedies, which she was able to print in large quantities. In this way Lady Grace spread medical ideas and knowledge to a wider reading public.

SOURCE 2

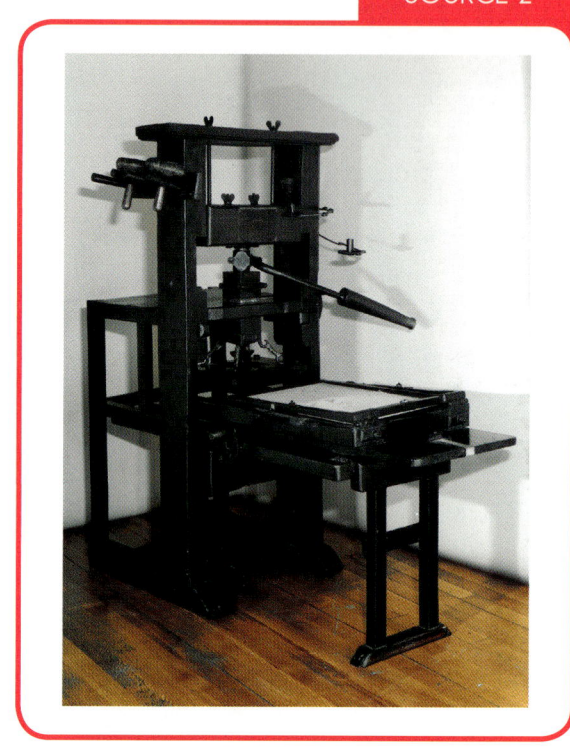

An early 18th century wooden printing press. This press follows a design that was in use by 1500 and persisted until the 1820s. The first British printer, William Caxton, would have used a similar press

TASKS

1. What can you learn about the Renaissance printing press from Source 2?
2. How important do you think the printing press was to the development of medical knowledge? Explain your answer.
3. Describe the contribution of Lady Grace Mildmay to the spread of medical knowledge.

Voyages of discovery

As part of this renewed interest in learning, people wanted to find out more about other parts of the world. In the late fifteenth and early sixteenth centuries, Spanish and Portuguese sailors had made long voyages of exploration. They had reached India, discovered the New World of the Americas, and brought back great wealth to their countries.

Voyagers like Christopher Columbus, who discovered America in 1492, brought new ideas, herbs, plants and medicines back to Europe. When Columbus had sailed westwards from Spain in 1492, he thought that he had landed in Asia and that he had discovered a new, westward route to the Spice Islands. At this time, spices were in great demand. Expensive spices were used more often for preparing medicines than for seasoning food. Portuguese explorers such as Bartholomew Diaz and Vasco da Gama explored the sea route to the Indian Ocean in search of these valuable spices.

SOURCE 3

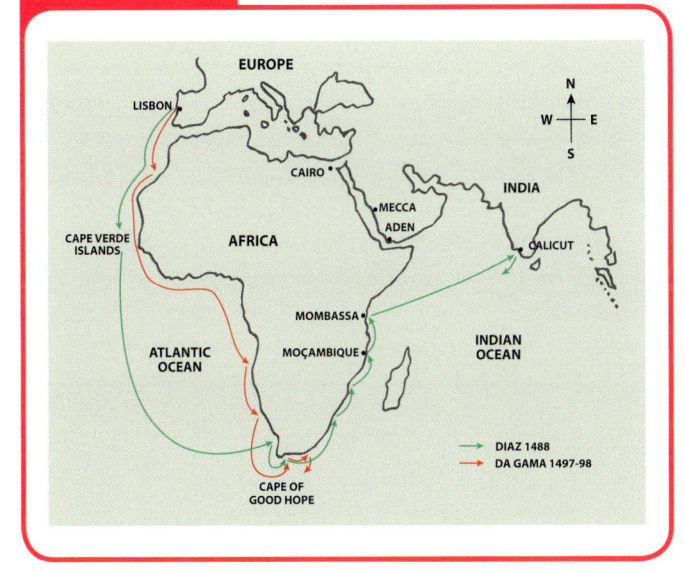

The voyages of Diaz and da Gama

By the mid sixteenth century there had been many more voyages of exploration and discovery and many supposedly valuable medicinal plants had been brought to Europe from the Americas, including

- Sassafras – dried bark of roots, used as a stimulant;
- Coca – dried leaves provided the source for cocaine;
- Sarsaparilla – dried roots were used as a tonic;
- Tobacco – claimed to be a wonder drug;
- Cinchona – indigenous South Americans used the bark of the cinchona tree; it is a source of quinine and was used to treat fevers, including malaria.

The use of these so-called medicinal plants was a by-product of the Renaissance. In their own way, these plants and the voyages that led to their discovery contributed to the development of medical knowledge at an important time in European history.

Renaissance art

The Italian Renaissance produced many brilliant and skilful artists and scholars. Changes in art at this time helped develop knowledge of the human anatomy. Before the Renaissance, knowledge of the human body was vague, as shown in the illustration in Source 4 and with the diagram of the 'Zodiac man' chart shown in Chapter 1.

SOURCE 4

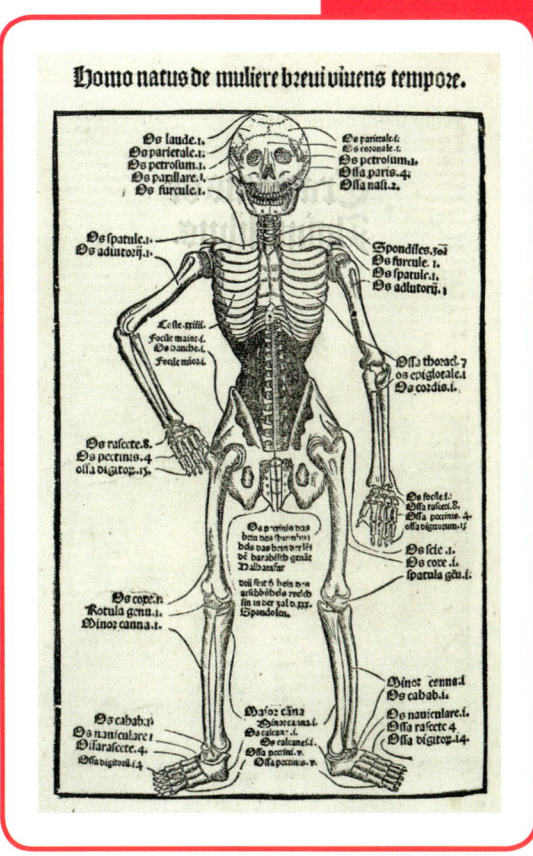

Medieval drawing of a human skeleton, c.1497

Two outstanding examples of these Renaissance artists were Michelangelo and Leonardo da Vinci. Both artists studied the human body in detail. Michelangelo studied the muscles and limbs and created sculptures of the human body, including his famous statue of David. He also painted the human body in great detail, as shown in the source below.

SOURCE 5

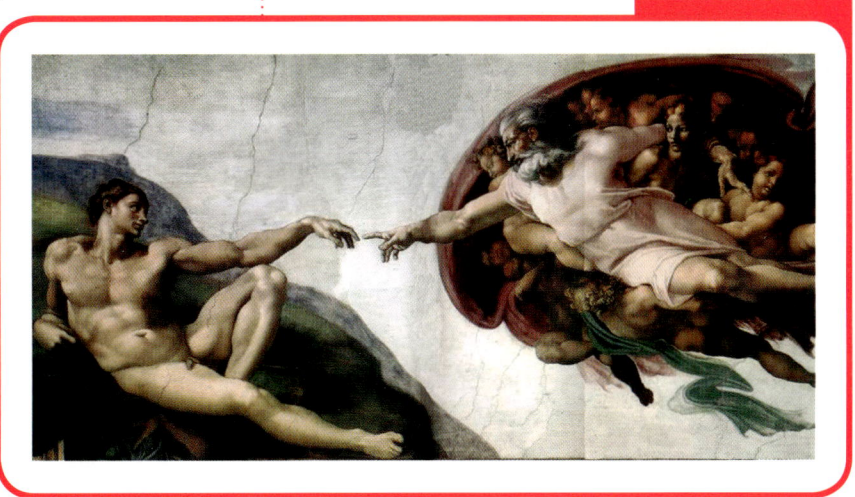

The Creation of Adam, painted by Michelangelo between 1508 and 1512

Leonardo da Vinci was an outstanding all-round genius. He was a painter, sculptor, architect and engineer. He studied how the human body worked and produced expertly detailed drawings of the human skeleton.

SOURCE 6

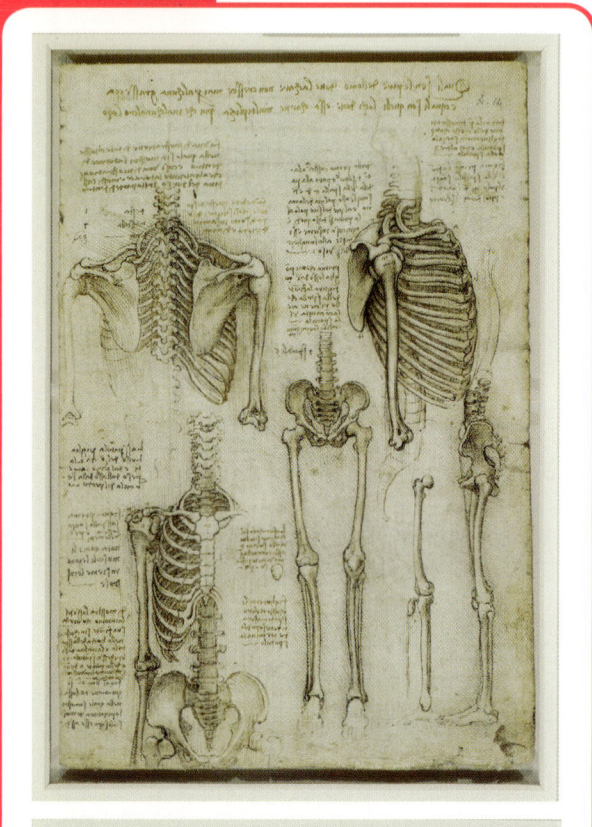

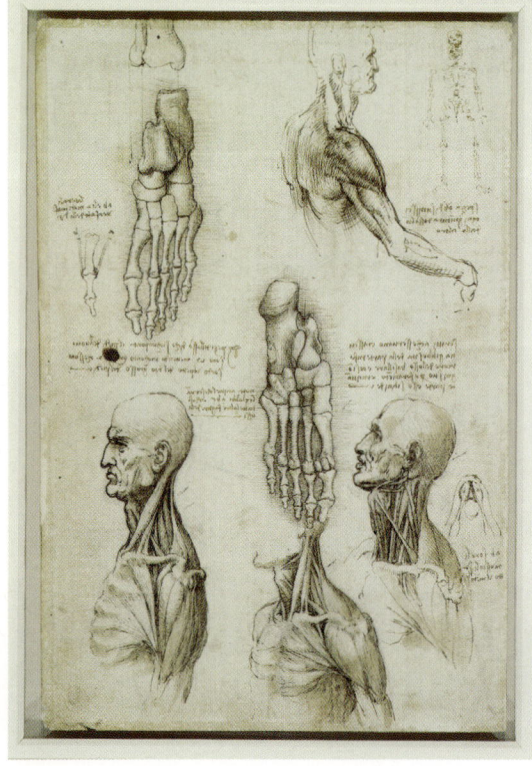

Leonardo da Vinci drawings of the human skeleton and the upper human body

Renaissance artists such as Michelangelo and da Vinci were able to draw the human body so accurately because they practiced dissection. The Church had banned dissections until the fourteenth century, but by about 1500 Renaissance artists had begun to perform their own dissections in order to study the human body in detail. The drawings that were produced as a result helped develop medical knowledge. They were included in medical books and, thanks to the invention of the printing press, were made widely available.

SOURCE 7

By 1500, ... with the establishment of the technology of printing, the images in medical works ... [were no longer] merely decorative ... they increasingly moved in the direction of naturalistic description. Through the medium of printing, woodcut illustrations became the bearers of detailed and exactly reproducible information

Historian Katharine Park, writing in the specialist book Western Medicine: An Illustrated History, *1997*

The invention of the printing press, the discovery of 'medicinal plants' in newly-discovered lands, the contribution of inspiring Renaissance artists and some very useful inventions such as the thermometer and the microscope, all combined to develop medical knowledge considerably in the sixteenth and seventeenth centuries. For over a thousand years, most Europeans had accepted the old ideas of writers such as Galen, but between 1500 and 1700 thinkers and teachers in universities began to challenge many of these ideas and put forward new ones of their own.

TASKS

1. What does Source 3 tell you about the search for spices?
2. Describe how Renaissance art helped to develop medical knowledge.
3. Which of the Renaissance ideas above do you think was the most important for the development of medical knowledge? Explain your answer fully.

IMPORTANT DEVELOPMENTS IN MEDICAL KNOWLEDGE

The Renaissance had encouraged people to develop new ideas. It also encouraged people to question old ideas. Paracelsus (1493-1541) is an example of a typical Renaissance man. He challenged existing ideas and put forward new ones and inspired others to do the same.

In 1523 Paracelsus became a lecturer at Basel University in Switzerland. The first thing that he did before he lectured was to burn the books of Galen. He said to his students:

> "You after me, … *Galenus* … You after me, not I after you. … I will be monarch, and mine the monarchy …
> I am exposing such a longwinded lie … I have cast … [Galen's] books into the St. John's Day fire …
>   My shoestrings are more learned than your *Galenus*"

From *Paracelsus: Theophrastus Bombastus von Hohenheim, 1493-1541: Essential Theoretical Writings*, edited and translated by Andrew Weeks, 2008, pp.75, 77, 79, 81, 97

No one had dared to criticise Galen like this before. Paracelsus made men question medical ideas and look for answers themselves. He insisted on observation and experience. Galen had said that diseases were caused by an imbalance of the four humours and that they would be cured by bloodletting and purging. Paracelsus believed that disease attacked from outside the body and he devised mineral remedies with which he thought the body could defend itself.

SOURCE 8

Paracelsus was … the most original medical theoretician of Renaissance Europe, in a period when medical creativity … was focused overwhelmingly on problems of practice and therapeutics. For the traditional Galenic and medieval model of physiology and illness, focused on complexional and humoral imbalance … Paracelsus substituted a model based on alchemical principles, which took the elements salt, sulphur, and mercury as the fundamental causal entities in both healing and disease.

Historian Katharine Park, writing in the specialist book Western Medicine: An Illustrated History, *1997*

Paracelsus still held on to some traditional ideas. For example, his work contained elements of magic, such as using a **talisman** to cure diseases. However, his criticisms of Galen and his ideas on observation and experience led medical thinking towards a more scientific approach. At the time, many doctors rejected his ideas because he had dared to challenge such long-held views. Even so, there were some individuals who were brave enough to build upon Paracelsus' radical new ideas and develop a more evidence-based approach to medicine.

Three of the most outstanding Renaissance thinkers who followed on in the tradition of Paracelsus were Andreas Vesalius, Ambroise Paré and William Harvey.

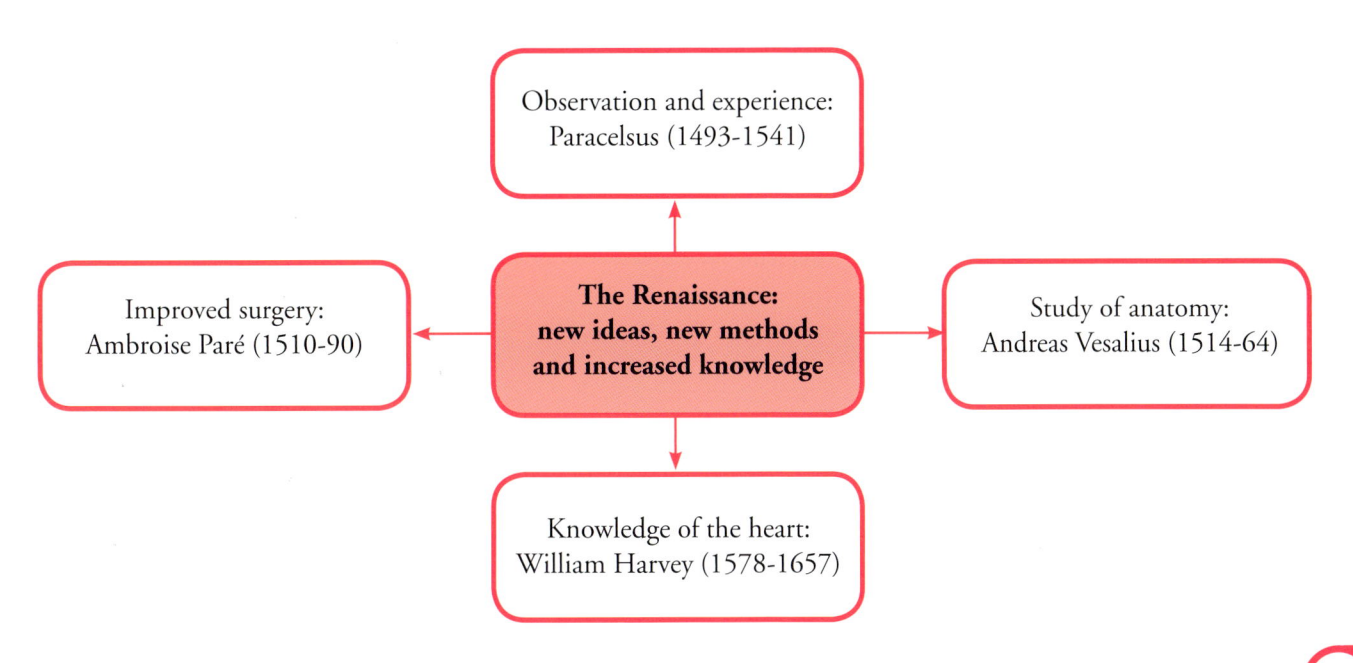

The Renaissance: new ideas, new methods and increased knowledge
- Observation and experience: Paracelsus (1493-1541)
- Improved surgery: Ambroise Paré (1510-90)
- Study of anatomy: Andreas Vesalius (1514-64)
- Knowledge of the heart: William Harvey (1578-1657)

Andreas Vesalius (1514-1564)

SOURCE 9

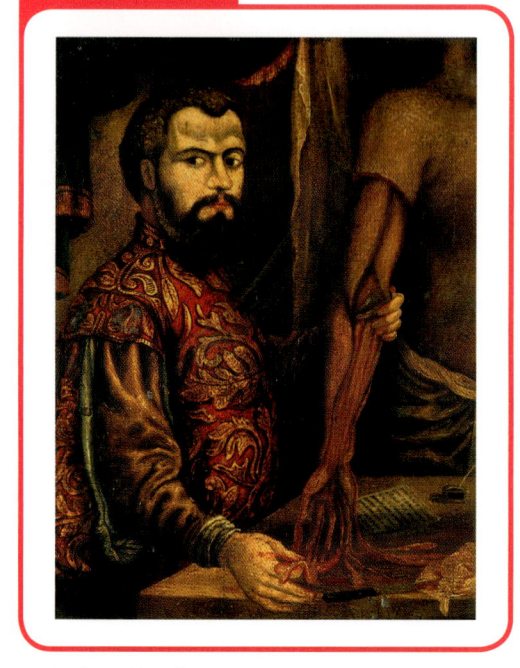

Andreas Vesalius

SOURCE 10

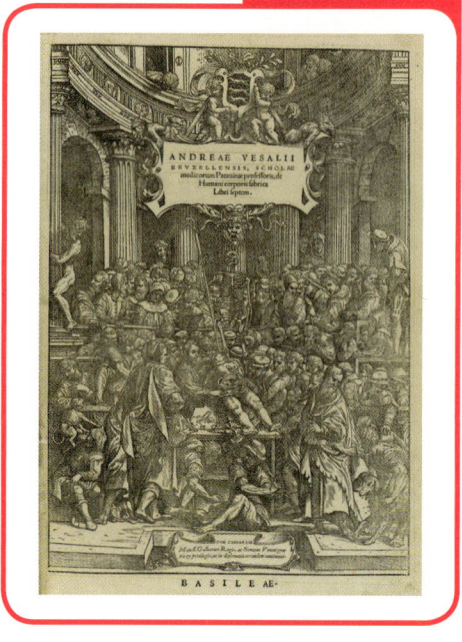

An artist's impression of Vesalius carrying out a dissection c.1543

Vesalius was born in Brussels, in modern-day Belgium. He studied medicine in Paris, where he learned a great deal about the human anatomy by examining skeletons from a cemetery in the city. He was later given the bodies of executed criminals to dissect. He also met Renaissance artists, who were studying skeletons and dissecting human bodies in order to make their paintings more realistic, and discussed with them details of the human anatomy.

Vesalius was a brilliant student and he became professor of anatomy at Padua University at the age of just 23. Hundreds of students would pack the lecture theatres to hear him deliver his lectures. Other lecturers would read aloud from the books of Galen while assistants carried out the dissections, but Vesalius performed the dissections himself. Like Paracelsus, Vesalius broke with the past when he told students to study the human body for themselves, instead of believing what they read in some of the old medical books written by ancient Greek and Arab writers. This was a major change – the questioning of old methods and the beginnings of a more investigative approach to medicine.

In 1543, Vesalius published his most famous book, *De humani corporis fabrica (On the fabric of the human body)*. Vesalius's book was the most important of all of the illustrated books of the time. It combined the Renaissance interest in anatomy with the skills of the Renaissance artists. It made full use of the new opportunities offered by the printing press and achieved immediate fame. Its excellent woodcuts were copied in books intended for general and professional readers, so that the study of anatomy flourished both in Italy and other parts of Europe. Vesalius was the first medical writer to realise the benefits of close links between the anatomist and the artist who had studied the human anatomy in detail, as Source 11 shows.

SOURCE 11

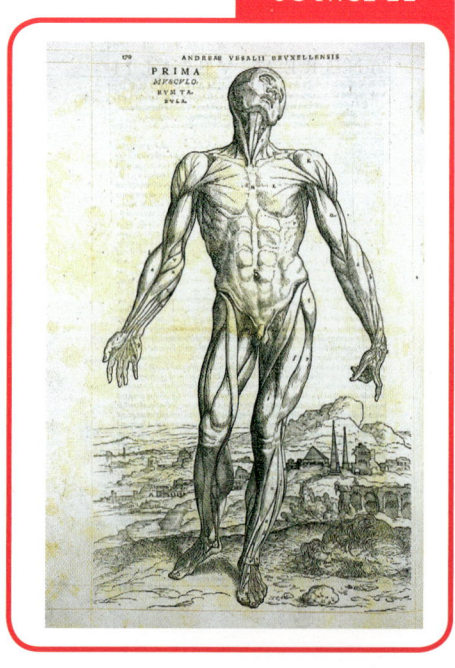

An anatomical drawing from Vesalius' On the fabric of the human body, 1543

Through his own work, Vesalius found that Galen had made mistakes. Galen had said that humans had the same number of bones in the spine as a monkey. Vesalius discovered that this was incorrect. He also found other mistakes that Galen had made and explained these in his book.

> "In most animals the jaw consists of two bones joined together … In man, however, the jaw is a single bone … Yet Galen and many other experts in dissection after Hippocrates asserted that the jaw is not a single bone"

From On the Fabric of the Human Body, Book 1: The Bones and Cartilages, *trans. by William Frank Richardson, 1998*

Older doctors and surgeons at Padua University opposed Vesalius and actually made fun of his ideas. They may have been jealous of his success at such a young age, but they were also angry that he had dared to suggest that Galen might be wrong.

Partly because of this opposition Vesalius left Padua to work as physician to Emperor Charles V. In 1555 he became physician to Charles' son, King Philip II of Spain. He died in 1564, on the return journey from a pilgrimage to Jerusalem.

SOURCE 12

The importance of Vesalius

Before Vesalius: doctors believed that the books of Galen and other ancient doctors were completely accurate and contained all the knowledge they needed. Therefore there was no need to learn more about anatomy by dissecting human bodies.

After Vesalius: Vesalius showed that Galen was wrong in some important details of anatomy. He believed that this was because Galen had to rely on dissecting animals. He said it was vital that doctors dissect human bodies to find out about the human structure and exactly how it works. He said doctors needed to test Galen's ideas instead of accepting them uncritically.

Historians I. Dawson and I. Coulson, writing in Medicine and Health through Time: *an SHP development study, 1996*

Vesalius' book and methods marked the beginning of a new era in medical knowledge, which was to continue as the Renaissance period progressed. His new approach to the study of anatomy laid the foundations for an increasingly scientific approach to medicine.

TASKS

1. Explain why Paracelsus was important in the development of medical knowledge.
2. Why was Vesalius' *On the fabric of the human body* important?
3. Describe how traditional ideas on medical knowledge changed because of Andreas Vesalius.
4. Study Source 11. What links this with Renaissance art?

Ambroise Paré (c.1510–1590)

SOURCE 13

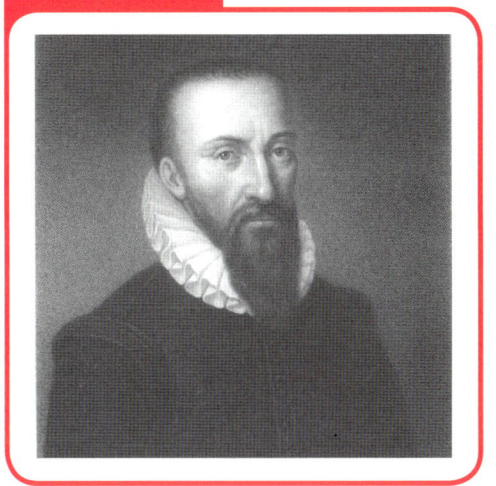

Ambroise Paré

Ambroise Paré changed people's ideas about surgery in the same way as Vesalius changed people's ideas about anatomy. Paré was born near Laval in France in 1510 and at a young age served as an apprentice to his brother, who was a barber – at this time barbers rather than physicians carried out surgery. He then went on to study at the Hôtel-Dieu Hospital in Paris and, after becoming a barber surgeon, joined the French army in 1536 as a regimental surgeon.

Paré gained his medical experience from the many wars in which France was involved during this time. He spent many years on campaign, treating sword and gunshot wounds. Source 14 shows where typical battlefield wounds were likely to be located.

SOURCE 14

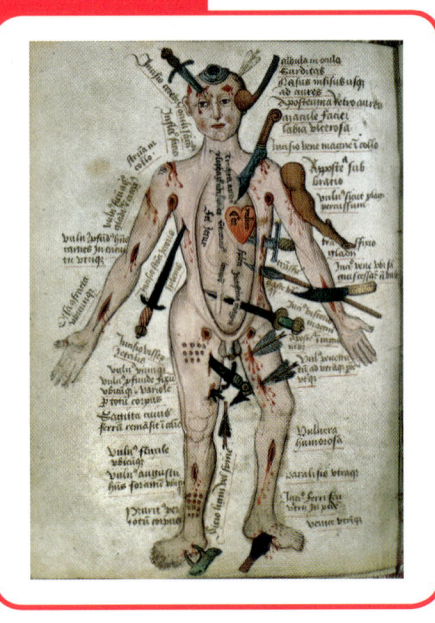

Wound man, *mid 15th Century*

At this time doctors thought that the formation of pus was a normal part of healing, rather than a sign that the wound was infected. A substance called a 'digestive' would be applied, and this was believed to break down matter in the wound (such as dead tissue) to pus, which would then be discharged taking any unwanted material with it. However, it was thought that gunshot wounds were poisoned by the gunpowder used in the **arquebus** to fire the ball, and the traditional way of treating these wounds was to **cauterise** them with boiling oil as quickly as possible. This method was painful and very dangerous and the wounds were always very inflamed and often became infected afterwards. On one occasion, Paré was unable to treat a gunshot wound in the usual way:

SOURCE 15

I ran out of oil and was **constrained** to apply a digestive made of egg yolk, oil of roses and turpentine. That night I could not sleep easily thinking that by the default in cautery I would find the wounded to whom I had failed to apply the said oil dead of poisoning ... Beyond my hopes I found those on whom I had put the digestive dressing feeling little pain from their wounds which were not swollen or inflamed, and having spent quite a restful night. But the others, to whom the said oil had been applied, I found fevered, with great pain and swelling around their wounds.
From then I resolved never again so cruelly to burn poor men wounded with arquebus shot.

From I. M. L. Donaldson's translation of part of Les Oeuvres de M. Ambroise Paré *of 1575*

During his time as an army doctor, Paré gained more knowledge about how to treat wounds. This included a method of stopping patients bleeding after an **amputation**. The traditional method was to press a red-hot iron, called a cautery, against the stump of the limb. This sealed the blood vessels and stopped the patient bleeding to death, but was exceedingly painful.

Paré tied threads, called ligatures, around the blood vessels to close them up. These ligatures proved to be a very effective and much less painful way of stopping the bleeding. Although the idea was not totally new it showed that Paré was prepared to try something different. He was quite exceptional in his willingness to experiment, which was very unusual for the sixteenth century.

Paré eventually retired from the army. He became a successful surgeon in Paris and from 1552 served under four different French kings. Like Vesalius before him, Paré was able to take advantage of the opportunities offered by the printing press to publish his work. In 1545 he published his observations on treating gunshot wounds and this little book was soon translated from French into several other languages and very rapidly led to a permanent change in the way these wounds were treated. In 1564, he published his *Treatise on Surgery*, and, in 1575, he collected all his observations together into *Les Oeuvres de M. Ambroise Paré (The Works of Mr Ambroise Paré)*. The book was written in French but was soon translated into Latin and other languages. It had a major impact on the treatment of wounds, on amputations and on the setting of fractures.

Paré developed an enquiring approach to his work and even turned his attention to the 'bezoar stone', which was said to have the power to counteract any kind of poison. Paré believed that this was impossible and was given the opportunity to prove this in 1564-5 whilst working as surgeon to the king. A cook was condemned to be hanged after being caught stealing silver. He was offered the alternative of being poisoned and immediately given an antidote, powdered bezoar stone, and promised that he would be set free if he survived. He readily accepted this alternative. The stone did not work and the cook died in severe pain several hours later. Paré had disproved a long-held view through the scientific method of experimentation and observation. Before his death in 1590, Paré also experimented with artificial limbs and developed new surgical tools and instruments.

SOURCE 16

The importance of Paré

Before Paré: wounds were treated by pouring boiling oil onto them. Doctors believed this would help them to heal. They stopped a wound bleeding by sealing it with a red-hot iron. This was called cauterising.

After Paré: Paré discovered that wounds healed more quickly if boiling oil was not used. Instead he put simple bandages onto wounds. He also stopped cauterising wounds. Instead he tied the ends of arteries using … thread.

Historians I. Dawson and I. Coulson, writing in Medicine and Health through Time: an SHP development study, *1996*

Many historians regard Paré as 'the father of modern surgery'. Like Vesalius before him, he was willing to experiment and find things out for himself. The changes introduced by Vesalius and Paré contributed greatly to developments in medical knowledge.

William Harvey (1578–1657)

SOURCE 17

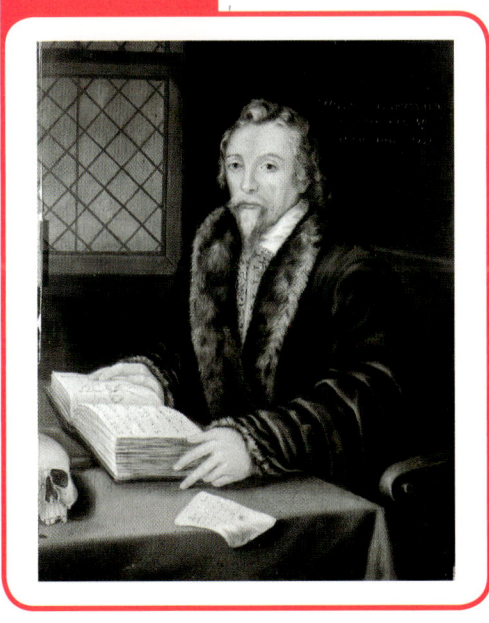

William Harvey

William Harvey was born at Folkestone in Kent and studied medicine at the universities of Cambridge and Padua. He worked as a doctor and then as a lecturer in anatomy. Like Vesalius and Paré, Harvey relied on observation and experiment to increase his knowledge. This led him to discover that the heart pumped blood around the body in a continuous loop.

The idea that the heart was a pump had been suggested almost two thousand years before Harvey's time, but it had not been possible to prove the theory. The fact that the heart acted like a pump was important to the understanding of blood flow. Harvey dissected live, cold-blooded animals in order to study the movements of each muscle in the heart. He dissected human bodies to build up a detailed knowledge of the heart. He pushed thin rods down the veins, proving that the blood flowed in one direction. He measured the amount of blood moved by each heartbeat and calculated how much was in the human body.

Harvey had built on the work of Italian artists that he had studied at the University of Padua. He presented detailed evidence in support of his conclusion that blood circulated through the arteries and veins, eventually returning to the heart, rather than simply flowing from the heart and liver to the furthest parts of the human body. Harvey published his findings in his book *Exercitatio Anatomica de Motu Cordis et Sanguinis in Animalibus (An Anatomical Study of the Motion of the Heart and of the Blood in Animals)* in 1628.

SOURCE 18

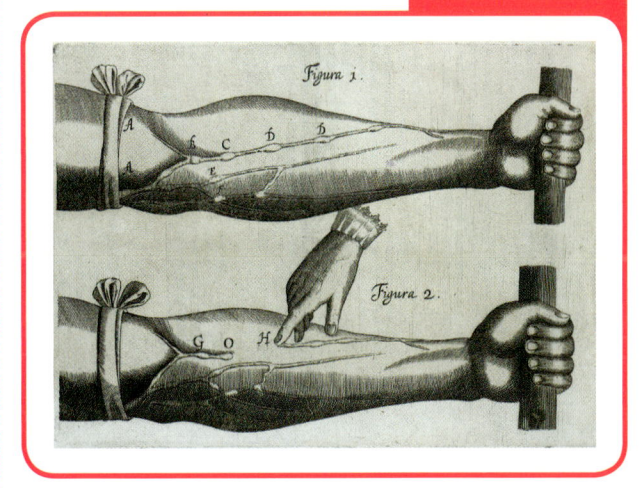

A drawing from Harvey's Anatomical Study

Harvey used the drawing in Source 18 to explain an experiment he carried out to prove that the blood will only travel in one direction through the veins. He said that if the upper arm is bandaged, as at A in Figure 1, the valves (G, O, H in Figure 2) show up as nodules, or small lumps, on the vein. If the finger is pushed along the vein from one valve to the next (e.g. from B to C or C to D in Figure 1) away from the heart, the section of vein between the valves will be emptied of blood. It will stay empty until the finger is taken off the valve, proving that blood will only flow in one direction.

Harvey's book increased people's understanding of how the body worked. In true Renaissance style, he had used investigative methods to show that blood travelled away from the heart through the arteries and back to the heart through the veins and that it travelled in a loop. William Harvey undoubtedly expected that his theories would be challenged because he opposed Galen's teachings, which suggested that blood moved from one side of the heart to the other through holes in the **septum**. Harvey's investigations had shown that there were no holes in the septum.

SOURCE 19

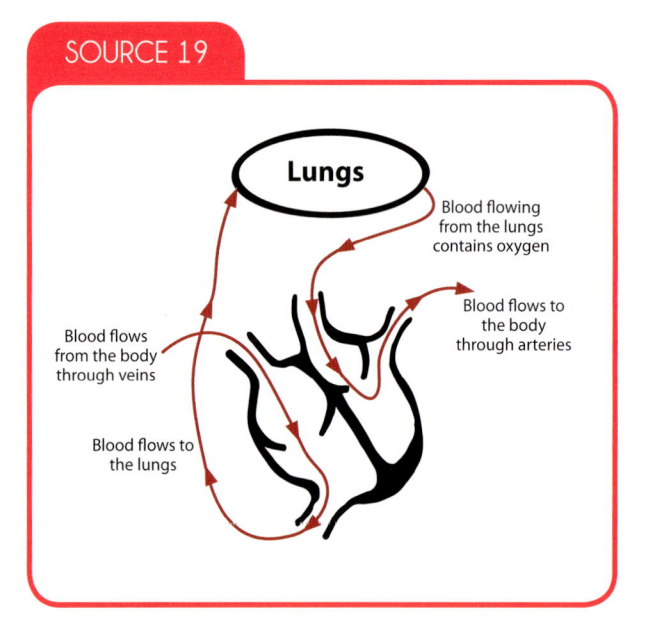

Diagram showing Harvey's ideas on the circulation of the blood

William Harvey became physician to two English kings, James I and Charles I. After the death of Charles I in 1649, Harvey returned to work in London. His work on the circulation of the blood remains his greatest contribution to the field of medicine.

SOURCE 20

The importance of Harvey

Before Harvey: many doctors still believed in Galen's idea that new blood was constantly being manufactured in the liver to replace blood that was burnt up in the body in the same way as wood is burnt by fire. This idea had been challenged by a number of doctors but no one had proved exactly how the blood moved around the body.

After Harvey: Harvey showed that blood flows around the body, is carried away from the heart by the arteries and returns to the heart in veins.
He proved that the heart acts as a pump, recirculating the blood[,] and that blood does not burn up[,] so no other organ is needed to manufacture new blood.

Historians I. Dawson and I. Coulson, writing in Medicine and Health through Time: an SHP development study, *1996*

The work of Vesalius, Paré and Harvey helped considerably in the advancement of medical knowledge. Their work was linked to earlier traditions but they had built on those traditions. Through a more scientific approach of observation and experimentation they had taken medical knowledge to a point from which there would be dramatic changes.

TASKS

1. Describe the changes that Paré brought to surgery.
2. In what ways did Harvey disagree with Galen?
3. Use Source 19 to describe the circulation of the blood, in your own words.
4. Describe how Harvey changed people's understanding of the working of the heart.

Examination practice

This section provides guidance on how to answer Question 1(b), 2(b) and 3(b) from Unit 3. The question asks you to describe, and it is worth 4 marks.

Question 1(b), 2(b), 3(b) – the understanding of a key feature through the selection of appropriate knowledge

Describe the work of William Harvey in the seventeenth century.

[4 marks]

Tips on how to answer

- Make sure that you only include information that is **directly relevant**.
- Jot down your initial thoughts, **making a brief list** of the points you intend to mention.
- After you have finished your list, try to put the points into **chronological order** by numbering them.
- It is a good idea to start your answer **using words from the question**, e.g. 'William Harvey's work in the seventeenth century …'
- Try to include **specific factual details** such as dates, events, the names of key people and important ideas. The more informed your description, the higher the mark you will receive.
- Aim to write a **good-sized paragraph**.

Response by candidate one

Harvey showed that blood circulated around the body. He also proved how our hearts work. They work 'like a pump' by pumping blood around the body. He wrote a book about his work.

Examiner's comment

This is a very generalised answer with weak points made. There is a lack of factual detail. This is a Level One answer, which would score half marks (2 marks).

Response by candidate two

Motion of the Heart (4), Cambridge and Padua (1), dissections (2), heart a pump (5), circulation (6), disproved Galen (7), physician to kings (3)

William Harvey studied medicine in both Cambridge and Padua universities. He carried out dissections on cold-blooded animals to find out how the muscles of the heart worked and he dissected human bodies in order to find out details about the human heart. He worked as a physician for King James I and for King Charles I and then published his ideas in *An Anatomical Study of the Motion of the Heart and of the Blood in Animals* in 1628. He proved an earlier theory that the heart is a pump, re-circulating blood around the human body. He showed that as blood flows around the body, it is carried away from the heart by arteries and returns to the heart in veins. William Harvey disproved the earlier ideas of Galen and he was a true representative of the new thinking of the Renaissance period.

Examiner's comment

This is a very detailed and accurate description of the work of William Harvey in the seventeenth century. The candidate has given prior thought to the details needed for the answer and has clearly identified the relevant factors, which have been placed in correct chronological order. These have been presented in a way that shows clear understanding. This is a full Level Two answer, worth the maximum 4 marks.

Now you have a go

Describe the work of Ambroise Paré in the sixteenth century.

[4 marks]

CHAPTER 3

HOW MUCH PROGRESS HAS BEEN MADE IN MEDICAL KNOWLEDGE FROM THE NINTEENTH CENTURY TO TODAY?

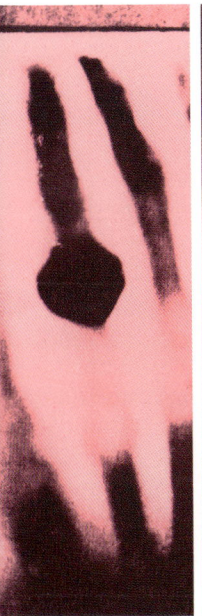

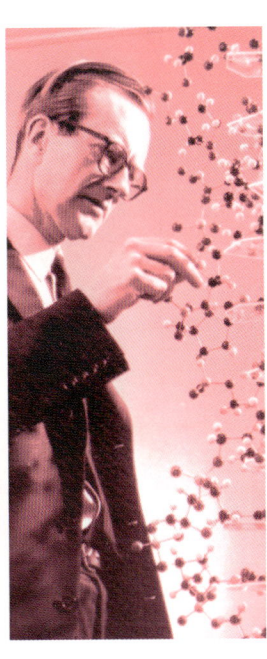

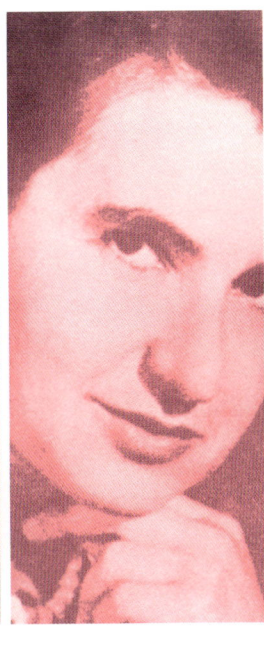

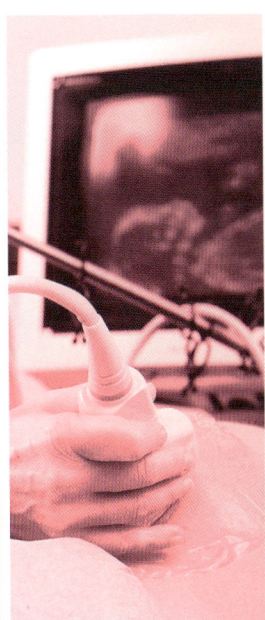

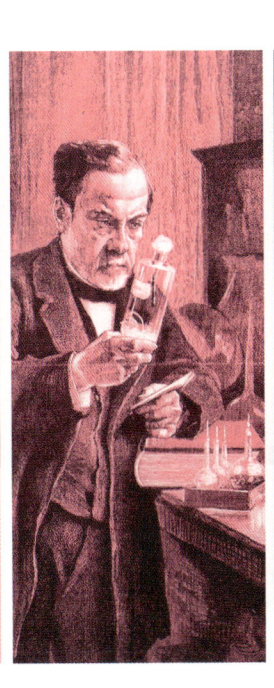

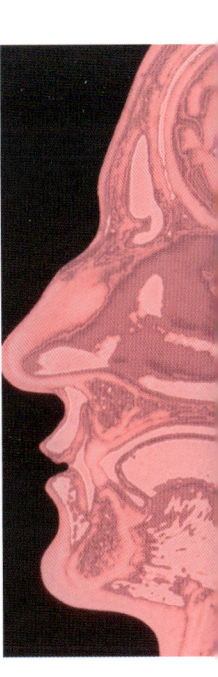

WORK ON THE GERM THEORY

From Harvey's work on the circulation of the blood in 1628 to Pasteur's Germ Theory in the 1860s, medical knowledge changed slowly but dramatically. The discoveries of the Renaissance period were a vital part of medical history and they were the foundation on which later scientists built their research. However, this did not lead to immediate improvements in people's health and life expectancy, as new and better ways of treating illnesses were yet to be found.

When someone became ill in the eighteenth and nineteenth centuries, they were still treated using the same traditional methods that had been used for hundreds of years. However, some important changes were occurring. There were more doctors and they were better trained. There were also **dispensaries** to provide cheap medicines for the poor. Moreover, by the 1860s, understanding of disease had reached a turning point.

It had been believed for centuries that there was a link between dirt and disease but no one had been able to prove this. During the Great Plague of London in 1665 people would carry strong smelling herbs around to overcome the fumes that they thought spread the plague. In the early nineteenth century, it was still popularly believed that **miasma**, or bad air, was responsible for spreading diseases, as poisonous fumes given off from rubbish and decaying matter were blown from one place to another. The fact that germs caused disease was yet to be proved.

In the late seventeenth century stronger and better microscopes led to the discovery that food and animal intestines, for example, contained tiny organisms, or micro-organisms. Further scientific experimentation then led to the claim in 1861 that certain types of micro-organisms, called germs, cause disease. This was known as the 'Germ Theory' and was very controversial when Louis Pasteur first announced it. Today it is an essential part of modern medicine and has led to innovations such as antibiotics and hygienic practices.

SOURCE 1

The ... idea that micro-organisms, 'germs', were responsible for many common, often fatal, diseases, such as diphtheria, measles, tetanus, typhoid, and cholera, gained ... acceptance from the work of many people. Foremost among these were the French chemist Louis Pasteur (1822-95) and the German pathologist Robert Koch (1843-1910), often regarded as the fathers of bacteriology.

Historian E. M. Tansey, writing in the specialist book Western Medicine: An Illustrated History, *1997*

Louis Pasteur

Louis Pasteur was born in eastern France where his father was a poor tanner. He was persuaded to go to Paris for his education and eventually gained his doctorate from the École Normale. In 1854, he was made professor of chemistry at the University of Lille, where he became interested in micro-organisms. He was asked to help a brewing company find out why the beer in their barrels was going bad. This problem was affecting both the brewing industry and the wine industry throughout France. With the aid of a microscope, Pasteur discovered that a particular micro-organism was growing in the brewing liquid. He developed a theory that these germs (so-called because the micro-organisms were germinating, or growing) were the cause of the problem and showed how to kill them by boiling and then cooling the beer. Today this process is called pasteurisation.

Pasteur went on to discover that micro-organisms were also responsible for turning milk and wine sour. He wanted to know from where these micro-organisms came.

SOURCE 2

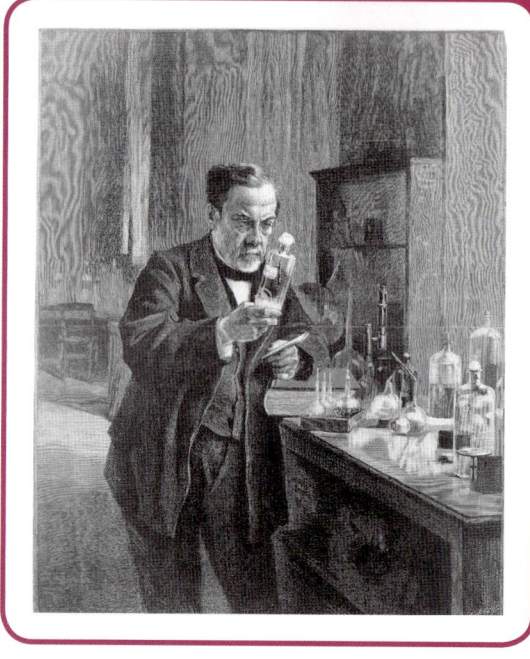

Louis Pasteur at work in his laboratory

Where did micro-organisms come from?

The old theory: spontaneous generation

The new theory: the germ theory

From the time of the ancient Romans to the late eighteenth century, it was believed that some living things grew spontaneously from non-living matter. This appeared to occur mainly in decaying matter, as in the case of maggots in rotting meat. The theory was known as 'spontaneous generation'. Doctors believed that spontaneous generation was also responsible for the presence of germs in infected wounds. They were unaware that germs could enter a wound from the air.

In 1859 the French Academy of Science organized a contest to prove or disprove the theory of spontaneous generation once and for all. Pasteur devised an experiment based on methods used by earlier scientists to prove that micro-organisms, or germs, are everywhere and that the long-held idea was wrong. He then went on to prove that it is these micro-organisms that cause decay.

Pasteur's ideas	Experiment that proved his ideas
The air contains living organisms	He took sterile flasks out into the streets of Paris. He opened them briefly and then quickly sealed them again. He found that bacteria grew in the flasks.
Microbes are not evenly distributed in the air	He repeated his sterile flask experiment in several places, including on mountains. He found that the number of bacteria varied.
Microbes in the air cause decay	He filled two flasks, one with sterile air and the other with ordinary air. In the sterile flask, there was no decay. In the other flask, decay occurred as normal.
Microbes can be killed by heating	He heated material in a flask to make it sterile. He drove the air out and then sealed the flask. The flask remained sterile, even for a very long time afterwards.

Pasteur's next step was to link micro-organisms to disease. Until now many doctors still believed in the **miasma theory**, but Pasteur had different ideas. He stated that "the germs of microscopic organisms abound in the surface of all objects, in the air and in water: … wines, beer, vinegar, the blood, urine and all the fluids of the body undergo none of their usual changes in pure air" (*Germ Theory and Its Applications to Medicine*, Louis Pasteur, Prometheus Books, 1996).

He wondered if harmful germs could get into a body, grow rapidly and then cause disease. He soon had an opportunity to put this new theory to the test. During the 1860s a disease that was affecting silkworms was devastating the French silk industry and Pasteur was called in to investigate. He found that a particular micro-organism seemed to be causing the silkworms' disease. This micro-organism would have to be eliminated.

A further step forward in the development of this Germ Theory was to prove the link between bacteria and human disease. However, Pasteur was a scientist, not a doctor and he had carried out his early experiments with beer, wine and silkworms. It was a German doctor, Robert Koch, who took up the challenge of applying these ideas to humans and, through a series of experiments, proved that specific micro-organisms cause specific human diseases.

Robert Koch

Koch was born in Germany in 1843. After qualifying as a doctor he worked for a short while in the General Hospital in Hamburg before settling in general practice. He was interested in the idea that diseases are caused by living micro-organisms. During the 1870s he set up a laboratory in his small flat and, using a microscope given to him by his wife, he carefully studied anthrax, a disease that can kill both animals and humans.

Koch's research methods

- Koch extracted the germ, or bacterium, that was believed to cause anthrax from the spleens of farm animals that had died of the disease. He grew this, studied it, and then injected it into mice. After a time the mice developed anthrax and died. Mice that he injected with blood taken from healthy animals did not suffer from the disease.
- Koch then took blood from an infected mouse. He isolated the anthrax bacterium and grew it through several generations in the laboratory to check that it was still the same. He injected this into another mouse and found that

SOURCE 3

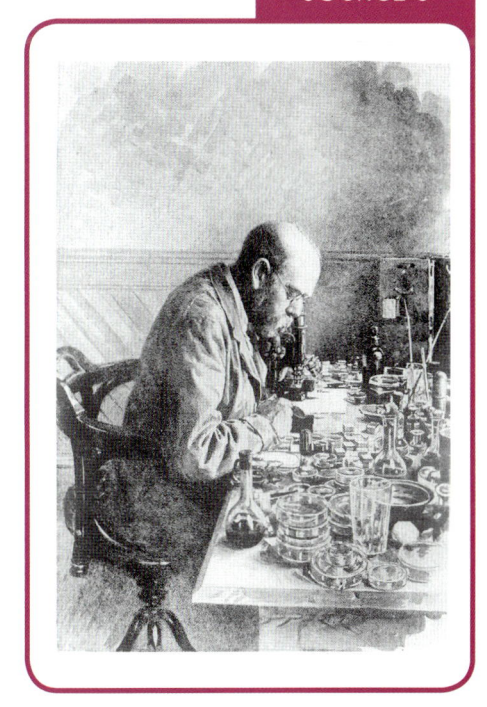

Robert Koch working in his laboratory

it too developed anthrax. He repeated this process many times and still had the same bacterium as at the beginning. Finally, Koch had proof that he had discovered the bacterium that caused the disease.

This systematic research provided a method that others could follow and enabled other scientists to identify the causes of different diseases. In 1876 Koch published a major work on the life cycle of the anthrax germ. He then went on to improve his techniques. In 1878, in his research into the bacterium that caused septicaemia (blood poisoning), he introduced the use of a purple dye, which coloured only certain bacteria, in order to see the bacterium more clearly.

Koch was appointed a member of the Imperial Health Bureau in Berlin in 1880 and was provided with a laboratory and a talented team of bacteriologists to carry on his research.

Robert Koch's achievements
- 1876 – isolated the germ that caused anthrax;
- 1878 – isolated the septicaemia germ;
- 1882 – isolated the tuberculosis germ;
- 1883 – isolated the cholera germ;
- 1885 – became professor of hygiene at the University of Berlin;
- 1891 – became the first director of the Prussian Institute for Infectious Diseases;
- 1905 – awarded the Nobel Prize for medicine.

Robert Koch's work in isolating germs made it possible to study them carefully and therefore to find out exactly what caused particular diseases. This made it easier to find a cure, although Koch himself did not discover the cures for the diseases that he studied.

Pasteur's continued efforts
Koch's success in isolating various bacteria spurred Pasteur into action again. Pasteur was a proud Frenchman and Koch was German. The Franco-Prussian War of 1870-71 had highlighted the great rivalry between these two countries. Pasteur now applied himself to what he considered the greatest challenge of all – finding cures for diseases.

Pasteur had thought a lot about Edward Jenner's work on smallpox and vaccination in the eighteenth century (see Chapter 4). He believed that smallpox was not the only disease that could be prevented through vaccination. However, as he did not know how vaccination worked, he had to continue his work by trial and error. In 1879 Pasteur was researching chicken cholera, a common disease in French farming at the time. He extracted the germ that caused the disease and went on to produce weaker forms. His team infected chickens with different strengths of solution made from the micro-organism to see if they worked.

During the summer of 1879, when the research was temporarily abandoned over the holidays, some chicken cholera solution was left unused in the laboratory. On returning to work, a member of the research team mistakenly injected chickens with the old germs that had been left exposed to the air. This led to an unexpected result: the chickens became immune to the disease. Pasteur was amazed at the discovery and called this method vaccination, to show his debt to Jenner. He had discovered a method of preventing the chicken cholera disease, but not of curing it.

In 1879 Pasteur turned his attention to anthrax. There was an anthrax epidemic in France and other parts of Europe at this time and the disease had killed a large number of sheep and cattle and was also attacking humans. After patient experimentation, Pasteur's team announced that they had produced a weak solution that they believed could immunise animals against anthrax. In 1881 the local agricultural society provided funds for Pasteur to attempt to immunise some farm animals in a public experiment.

SOURCE 4

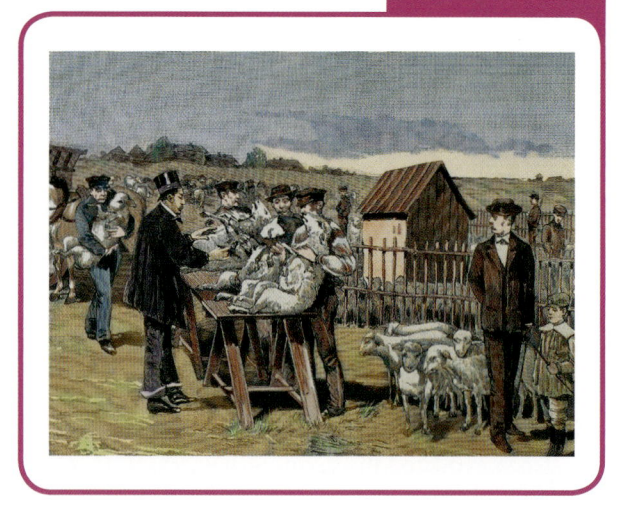

Pasteur vaccinating sheep against anthrax, 5 May 1881

The experiment was carried out with 60 animals on a farm in the small village of Pouilly-le-Fort, to the south of Paris in May and June 1881. Pasteur proceeded as follows:

SOURCE 5

On May 5, 1881, we used a Pravaz syringe to inoculate twenty-four sheep, one goat and six cows each with five drops **attenuated** anthrax. On May 17, we revaccinated these ... by more anthrax. While this microbe was also attenuated, it was more **virulent** than the anthrax used in the previous vaccination.

On May 31, we proceeded to inoculate these animals with the very virulent anthrax ... we inoculated the thirty-one vaccinated animals above [with the very virulent strain], and also twenty-four other sheep, one goat and four other cows, none of which had been exposed to this treatment previously. ...

With the inoculations completed, all the people present decided to meet again on Thursday June 2, 48 hours after the inoculations with the very virulent anthrax.

When the visitors arrived on June 2, they were astounded. The twenty-four sheep, the goat, and the six cows which had received the vaccinations of attenuated anthrax, all appeared healthy. In contrast, twenty-one sheep and the goat which had not been vaccinated had already died of anthrax; two other unvaccinated sheep died in front of the viewers, and the one remaining sheep died at the end of the day.

The unvaccinated cows had not died ... However [within 48 hours], the unvaccinated cows all showed significant **edema** at the place right behind the shoulder where they were inoculated. ... The temperature of these cows increased 3°C. The vaccinated cows did not show an elevation in temperature, swelling, or even the slightest loss of appetite.

From 'Summary Report of the Experiments Conducted at Pouilly-le-Fort, Near Melun, on the Anthrax Vaccination', by Louis Pasteur (with the collaboration of Mr Chamberland and Mr Roux), translated by Tina Dasgupta

Pasteu'r experiment was a complete success: the anthrax vaccine had worked and a method of preventing another disease had been discovered. The outcome was even reported in the British newspapers at the time.

In 1882, feeling confident with his methods, Pasteur turned his attention to another killer disease – rabies. Rabies is passed to humans from a bite by an infected animal, often a dog. After two years of careful research Pasteur developed a successful rabies vaccine, which brought him worldwide fame and began an era of **preventative medicine**.

Pasteur's achievements:
- He had proved that beer and wine went bad due to the presence of micro-organisms, or germs;
- He discovered how to eliminate germs from liquids through boiling and then cooling – a process later known as pasteurisation;
- He used Edward Jenner's practice of vaccination to prevent anthrax, once the bacterium that caused the disease had been isolated;
- He produced vaccinations for chicken cholera, diphtheria and rabies.

The first cures

Pasteur's vaccinations were able to prevent diseases, but not to cure them. However, the first cures were soon to follow on from the work of Pasteur and Koch. The German physiologist Emil Behring found that animals produced anti-toxins to fight harmful bacteria. In 1890, he took blood from an animal that had recovered from diphtheria, removed the clotting agents to create a serum (a clear liquid), and injected this into a patient who was suffering from diphtheria. The patient was cured.

Behring had used natural means to cure diphtheria. The search was now on to discover the first chemical cure. German physician Paul Ehrlich had joined Koch's research team at the Institute of Infectious Diseases in 1891. Koch had discovered that in some cases, dyes could stain certain bacteria and make them easier to see. However, he had been unable to make much progress in his research. Ehrlich was fascinated by dyes and he experimented with hundreds of different ones to see which bacteria they would seek out. This research led him to discover that the blood carries antibodies that kill particular germs. He called them 'magic bullets' because they found the micro-organisms they wanted to kill without harming others that the body needed.

Ehrlich realised that he could use dyes to carry drugs to certain tissues, without harming other tissues on the way. His team made an outstanding discovery in 1905 when they created Salvarsan, which cured syphilis. Medical knowledge was certainly increasing rapidly.

TASKS

1. What does Source 2 tell you about Pasteur's method of working?
2. Why was the germ theory a turning point in medical knowledge?
3. Write a short pragraph to describe Robert Koch's success in isolating germs.
4. Why was Pasteur's later work important?
5. Describe how the first cures were made possible by the work of Paul Ehrlich.

THE DEVELOPMENT OF SCANNING TECHNIQUES

The germ theory had been proved because of the work of some outstanding individuals. However, it was not only the contributions of these people that helped to develop medical knowledge. Sometimes war played a significant role. The German physicist Wilhelm Röntgen had discovered X-rays in 1895, and their possible use in medicine had been recognised immediately. However, during the First World War the use of X-rays became routine as doctors used them to find bullets and **shrapnel** that had become lodged inside the bodies of wounded soldiers.

The work of Wilhelm Röntgen

SOURCE 6

Perhaps the most extraordinary discovery [of the late nineteenth century] ... was that of X-rays in late 1895, the result of an unexpected observation by the physicist Wilhelm Röntgen (1845-1923). The potential of X-rays was recognized immediately, and they were rapidly integrated into hospital practice, heralding a move towards non-invasive diagnostic procedures that would grow throughout the twentieth century.

Historian E. M. Tansey, writing in Western Medicine: An Illustrated History, *1997*

Röntgen gained his doctorate from the University of Zurich in Switzerland before becoming a lecturer and later a professor at various German Universities. Whilst working at the University of Würzburg in 1895, he was studying the effects of passing a current through a gas at very low pressures in a glass tube. After covering the tube with black card in order to stop the light produced from escaping, Röntgen was amazed to find that unknown rays were passing through and lighting up the other side of the room. After investigating further, he found that the rays could also pass through wood, rubber and even human flesh, but not through bone or metal.

As he knew nothing about their properties, Röntgen called these mysterious rays X-rays. However, he was very aware of their potential importance. The X-ray photograph of his wife's hand that was published in his report in December 1895 was the first medical image showing the unseen world inside the human body. Röntgen's discovery caused great public excitement and had an immediate impact on medicine.

SOURCE 7

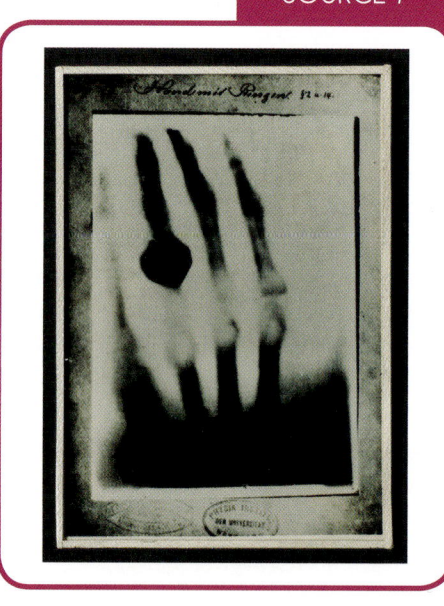

An X-ray image of the hand of Röntgen's wife

Within six months many hospitals had installed X-ray machines. However, it was the First World War that confirmed the importance of this new technology. More X-ray machines were quickly manufactured to meet the needs of wounded soldiers and installed in major hospitals all along the Western Front.

X-rays greatly improved the success rate of surgeons as they removed deeply lodged bullets and shrapnel from wounded soldiers. They also marked the beginning of **non-invasive surgery** and led to the development of further scanning techniques.

SOURCE 8

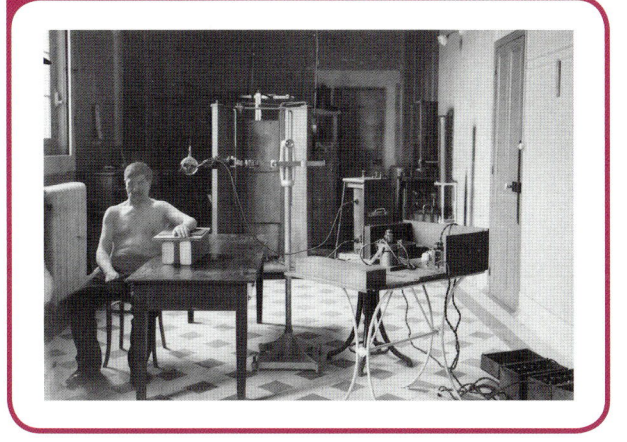

Performing an arm X-ray with the help of a portable X-ray machine, 1915

Modern scanning techniques

X-ray photography has allowed doctors to see inside the body without surgery. For this reason, it has been described as "perhaps the most extraordinary discovery of the late nineteenth century". Many more scanning methods have now been developed, such as ultrasound, magnetic resonance imaging (MRI), positron emission tomography (PET) and computerised tomography (CT). These provide powerful tools that enable specialist doctors to distinguish between what is normal and what is not inside the human body.

Ultrasound scans

SOURCE 9

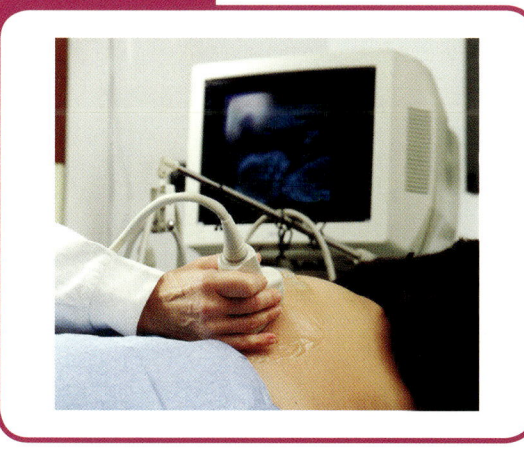

Ultrasound scanning is used to produce images of the foetus inside the womb

Ultrasound scanning, or imaging, developed from the 1950s. The technique involves exposing parts of the body to high frequency sound waves to produce pictures of what is inside. Unlike X-rays the process does not use radiation. Ultrasound scanning can provide 3-D images of the structure and movement of the body's internal organs, as well as blood flowing through vessels.

Ultrasound scanning is commonly associated with seeing pictures of an unborn foetus inside the womb. However, it can also help to diagnose a variety of conditions and assess organ damage following illness. It is used to help doctors to evaluate pain, swelling and infection and is a useful way of examining the body's internal organs. Ultrasound scanning is also used to guide procedures such as needle biopsies in which needles are used to extract sample cells from an abnormal area of the body for laboratory testing. This is done in cases of breast cancer and in diagnosing a variety of heart conditions.

MRI scans

The first MRI scan of a human body was carried out in 1977. An MRI scanner uses a strong magnetic field and radio waves to create computerised pictures of tissues, organs and other features inside the body.

Short bursts of radio waves are sent from the scanner to the body. Different signals are sent back from different body tissues: softer tissues can therefore be distinguished from harder tissues. A receiving device in the MRI scanner detects these signals, which are then transmitted to a computer where a picture is created.

The MRI scanner itself is a 1.5 m long tunnel, surrounded by a circular magnet. The patient lies on a bed that slides into the scanner. A receiving device, like an aerial, detects the tiny radio signals emitted from the body. The whole process is painless and usually takes between 15 and 40 minutes.

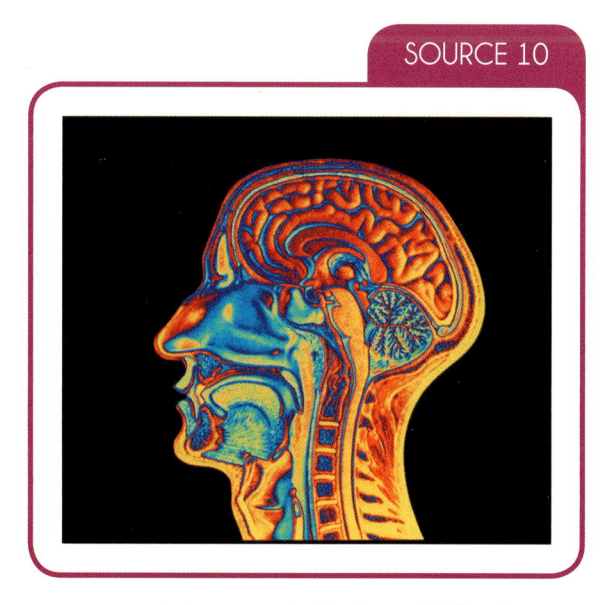

SOURCE 10

An image created during an MRI head scan

An MRI scan can take clear pictures of most parts of the human body. It is useful when other tests, like X-rays, do not give enough information. It is commonly used to get detailed pictures of the brain and spinal cord, in order to detect abnormalities and tumours. Even torn ligaments around joints can be detected by an MRI scan, and it is being used increasingly following sports injuries.

PET scans

SOURCE 11

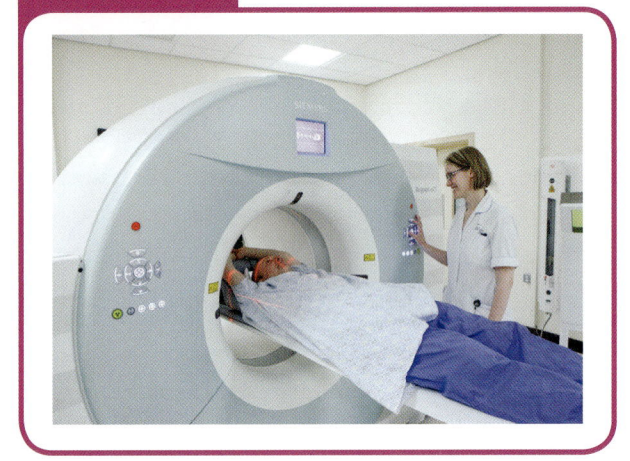

A PET scanner

A PET scan is a technique that produces a three-dimensional image of parts of the human body. This technique was first used effectively in the early 1970s.

A very small dose of radioactive chemical, called a **radiotracer**, is injected into the patient's body. This tracer travels through the body and is absorbed by the organs and tissues being studied. The patient is then moved into the PET scanner, a doughnut-shaped machine, as seen in Source 11, which detects and records the energy being given off by the tracer substance. With the aid of a computer, this energy is converted into three-dimensional pictures.

PET scanning is useful in detecting cancer, brain diseases and heart problems. The main difference between this and other scanning methods is that the PET scan reveals details of the cells of an organ or tissue. A PET scan can often detect cellular changes earlier than MRI or CT scans. Although PET scanning is non-invasive, it does involve exposure to radiation.

CT scans

A CT scanner is a special kind of X-ray machine. This type of scanner was introduced in the 1970s. Instead of sending a single X-ray through the body as with ordinary X-rays, several beams are sent at the same time from different angles. 'Tomography' means imaging by sections and this is what the CT scanner does: it takes images of the body in sections.

The patient slides into the CT scanner – a similar looking machine to that shown in Source 11. The X-rays from the beams emitted by the scanner are detected after they have passed through the body and their strength is then measured. Beams that have passed through less dense tissue like the lungs will be stronger, whereas beams that have passed through denser tissue such as bone will be weaker. A computer processes the results and a two-dimensional picture is shown on a monitor. British inventor Sir Godfrey Hounsfield, who was awarded the Nobel Prize for his work, developed the technique of CT scanning.

CT scans are much more useful than ordinary X-rays. They allow doctors to see inside the body in far greater detail. The information can be used to produce images that show what a surgeon will see during an operation. CT scanning has proved invaluable in pinpointing tumours and in planning treatment with radiotherapy. Scanning techniques have progressed enormously from 1895 when Wilhelm Röntgen first made his amazing discovery of X-rays. They have allowed doctors to increase their knowledge of the human body and to make huge advances in non-invasive surgery.

TASKS

1. How important was Röntgen's discovery of X-rays? Explain your answer fully.
2. Explain why the First World War was important for Röntgen's discovery.
3. Research the work of Sir Godfrey Hounsfield in the field of medicine.

DEVELOPMENTS IN GENETICS

Genetics is a branch of biology that studies heredity and genes. It tries to explain what genes are and how they work.

Modern genetics began towards the end of the nineteenth century. The word 'gene' was used for the first time in 1909, giving 'genetics' its name. Genes are the means by which living organisms inherit features from their ancestors: for example, children usually look like their parents because they have inherited their parents' genes. Genetics tries to identify which features are inherited and explain how these features are passed from one generation to the next.

Evidence was also found in 1909 that genes occur on chromosomes, which are rod-shaped structures in the nucleus of all living cells. A more detailed study of genetics began in the 1940s when it was shown that all genetic information was carried by a particular component of these chromosomes, called DNA (deoxyribonucleic acid). By the early 1950s the race was on to discover the structure of DNA, the so-called building block of life.

The discovery of DNA

By 1952 much was known about DNA, including its exclusive role as genetic material – the one substance that stores practically all the information needed to create a living thing. What was not yet known was what the DNA molecule looked like, or how it performed this amazing hereditary function. This would change within the course of a year.

SOURCE 12

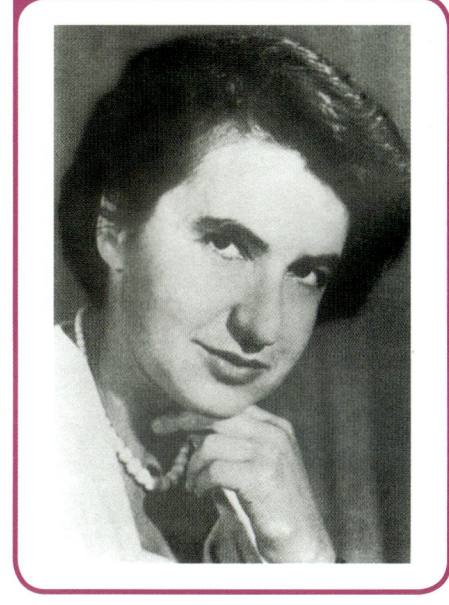

Rosalind Franklin

Rosalind Franklin (1920-58) was a British biophysicist and chemist. She worked in the Medical Research Council Biophysics Unit at King's College, London, researching the structure of DNA. Maurice Wilkins worked at the Unit with her. Using a technique called X-ray diffraction Franklin discovered that the DNA molecule consisted of an intertwined double helix of atoms.

At the same time, James Watson and Francis Crick were also researching the structure of DNA at Cambridge University. Unbeknown to Rosalind Franklin, Maurice Wilkins showed Watson and Crick the X-ray diffraction data that she had collected. This was the data they needed to complete their research, and in April 1953 Crick and Watson published an article called *Molecular Structure of Nucleic Acids: A Structure for Deoxyribose Nucleic Acid*. Here at last was an explanation of the structure of the DNA molecule – a double helix, or spiral staircase structure.

SOURCE 13

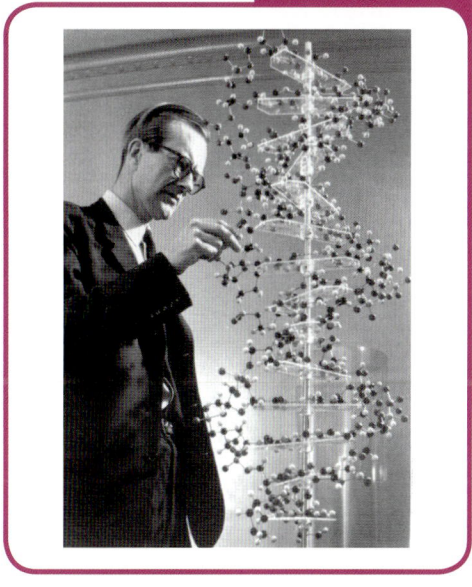

Maurice Wilkins with a model of the double helix

Watson and Crick's discovery helped to explain how DNA replicates and how hereditary information is coded in it. This set the stage for the rapid advancements in molecular biology that continue to the present day. Their discovery has been regarded as one of the principal medical triumphs since the Second World War and even as one of the most significant discoveries of the twentieth century. In recognition of their achievement, Watson, Crick and Wilkins were awarded the Nobel Prize for medicine in 1962 "for their discoveries concerning the molecular structure of nucleic acids and its significance for information transfer in living material". Rosalind Franklin had died in 1958, aged just 37. The Nobel Prize can only be awarded to living people.

SOURCE 14

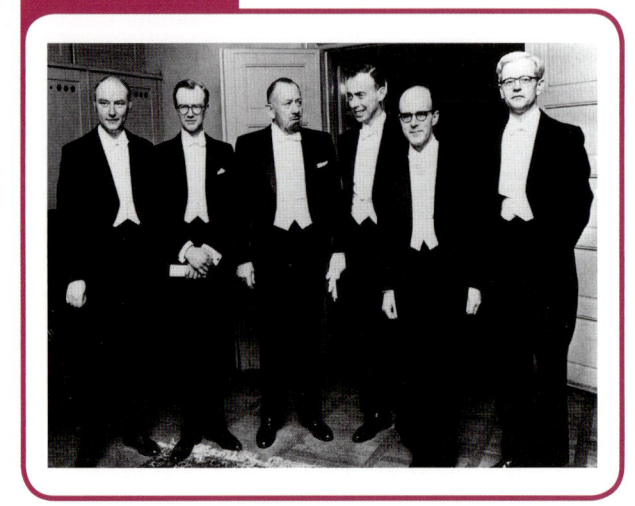

Francis Crick (left), Maurice Wilkins (2nd left) and James Watson (3rd right) pictured at the Nobel Prize ceremony, 1962

Continued developments in genetics

As a result of Watson and Crick's discovery, scientists have been able to identify that the causes of some illnesses are genetic. It is important to understand genetics in order to diagnose, prevent and treat **hereditary diseases**.

Some of the most recent breakthroughs are the use of DNA in crime cases, the determination of relatives and even the cloning of animals. Dolly the sheep was a Welsh Mountain sheep that lived for six years (1996-2003). She was cloned from a single cell of an adult sheep, proving that whole animals can be recreated artificially.

The discovery of the DNA molecule and the development of more powerful microscopes have enabled scientists to see not just the body's cells, but the chromosomes and genes within them. This, in turn, has led to genetic engineering, which started in the 1970s. Genes can now be manipulated to correct problems in a patient's body. For example, DNA can be made to produce the important protein insulin, which occurs naturally in most people, but is absent in those suffering from diabetes. Genetic engineering can also produce antibodies that seek out and destroy specific cells within the body.

James Watson became the first Director of the Human Genome Project in 1988. A genome is the full set of chromosomes and genes that an individual organism possesses. The project was based at the American National Institute for Health and was an international research project with the aim of mapping the human genome – the details of the entire sequence of genes in the human body (totalling some 50,000-100,000). The genome of each individual (except for identical twins and cloned organisms) is unique. The Human Genome Project was completed in 2003.

Conclusion

Medicine has advanced considerably since the late Middle Ages. From basic and sometimes superstitious ideas about drugs and potions, medical knowledge has developed at varying rates over the centuries, so that we now have an excellent understanding of the human body and the causes of illness. Future generations may take this knowledge even further, creating an understanding that is currently undreamt of.

TASKS

1. What is genetics?
2. Describe the role of Rosalind Franklin in the discovery of DNA.
3. Why has the discovery of the structure of DNA been important?
4. Do some research to find out more about Dolly the sheep. Briefly explain Dolly's importance.

Timeline

1. Construct a timeline of some of the major changes in the field of medicine from the Middle Ages to the present day.
2. Which change do you think was the most important? Explain your answer fully.

Essay question

Has the expansion of medical knowledge always been successful from the late Middle Ages to the present day?

[10 marks]

You may wish to discuss the following in your answer:
- *The impact of common ideas in the late Middle Ages;*
- *The influence of Renaissance ideas;*
- *Advances in knowledge such as the development of the germ theory;*
- *Developments in genetics;*
- *Any other relevant factors.*

(For advice on answering this question, see page 73)

Examination practice

This section provides guidance on how to answer Question 1(c), 2(c) and 3(c) from Unit 3. The question is worth 6 marks.

Question 1(c), 2(c), 3(c) – the understanding of change/continuity through the comparison of two sources and the use of own knowledge

Look at these two sources about developments in medical knowledge and answer the question that follows.

SOURCE A

Vesalius specialised in anatomy. He dissected human bodies to improve his medical knowledge. In 1543, his book *On the Fabric of the Human Body* was published, which included detailed drawings of the human anatomy.

A description of Andreas Vesalius' work

SOURCE B

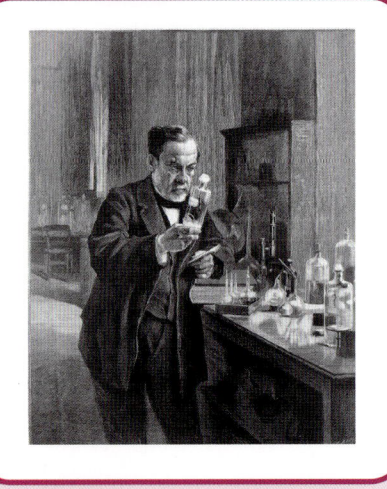

Louis Pasteur in his laboratory with a microscope on the bench beside him

Question

Use Sources A and B and your own knowledge to show how medical knowledge increased from the sixteenth to the nineteenth century.

[6 marks]

Tips on how to answer

This question asks you to identify change or lack of change (continuity) and to use your own knowledge to help describe and explain this, placing each source in context. To do this you need to:

- **Describe** what is in each source, making use of the caption written next to it.
- **Refer directly to each source**
  e.g. *Source A says… This contrasts with Source B, which shows…*

- Attempt to **cross-reference**, pointing out what is the same or different in each source.
- Remember to **include specific factual detail** from your own knowledge to help place each source in its historical context.
- If you only use your own knowledge and do not specifically refer to the sources you will not be given more than half marks.
- To reach the highest level you need to ensure that you have described and explained both sources, **focused on the key issue of change or continuity** and supported this with your own knowledge of the topic.

Response by candidate one

Vesalius studied anatomy, and people determined how you were ill by looking at the stars. Leonardo da Vinci drew the first accurate drawings of the human body. Harvey showed how blood circulated around our body and how our heart works. Paraclesus showed there are chemicals in our body. The biggest increase was when Pasteur discovered germs. But he couldn't have discovered this without knowing how the body worked.

Examiner's comment

The answer is based almost entirely on the candidate's own knowledge. The sources are implied but the answer is mostly descriptive. The candidate has identified what has changed but there is no specific mention of either Source A or Source B. The marks awarded will be confined to Level Two and would score 3 out of 6.

Response by candidate two

In Source A, it describes the work of Vesalius in his book 'Fabric of the Human Body'. Medical knowledge was increased due to the fact that Vesalius disproved the ideas of Galen. Anatomical ideas were fused with art to present detailed anatomical descriptions never seen before. Due to the printing press (Johannes Gutenberg, 1454), Vesalius's ideas could be shared amongst the scientific community and used to encourage more dissections and to give lectures to teach students.

Source B shows Louis Pasteur, the innovator of the germ theory. Germs were then considered to be causes of illness and the germ theory was established. Pasteur's work, along with Robert Koch's work, increased medical knowledge and led to cures and treatments for illnesses such as cholera, dysentery, tuberculosis and septicaemia. Microscopic study meant that more people considered studying bacteria in relation to medicine.

Examiner's response

The candidate has referred directly to both sources and has produced a structured and well-informed answer. There is an attempt to explain and analyse the content of both sources, expanding upon points through inclusion of own knowledge. There is no attempt at cross-referencing but there is a focus on change. The answer is not always well written but it matches most of the requirements for Level Three. It is worthy of being awarded 5 marks out of 6.

Now you have a go

Look at these two sources about scanning techniques and answer the question that follows.

SOURCE C

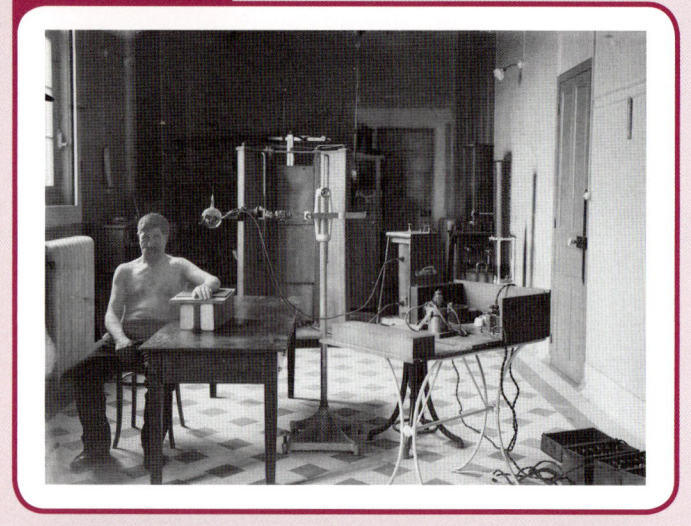

A portable X-ray machine used during the First World War

SOURCE D

An MRI scanner uses a strong magnetic field and radio waves to create pictures on a computer of features inside the human body. It is useful when other scanning methods, like X-rays, do not give enough information. An MRI scan can get detailed pictures of the brain and spinal cord, and detect abnormalities and tumours.

A description of an MRI scanner

Question

Use Sources C and D and your own knowledge to show how scanning techniques have changed over the past century.

[6 marks]

CHAPTER 4

HOW DID METHODS OF TREATING DISEASE IN WALES AND ENGLAND CHANGE FROM THE LATE MIDDLE AGES TO THE EIGHTEENTH CENTURY?

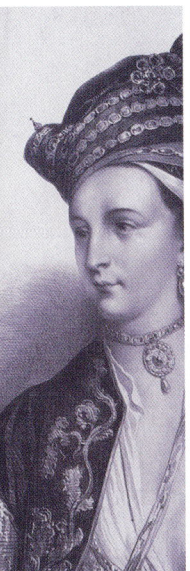

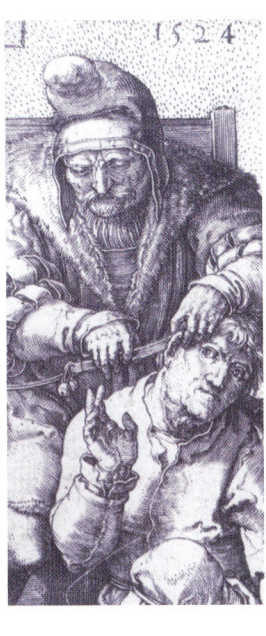

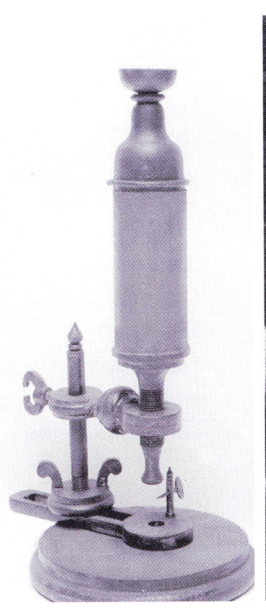

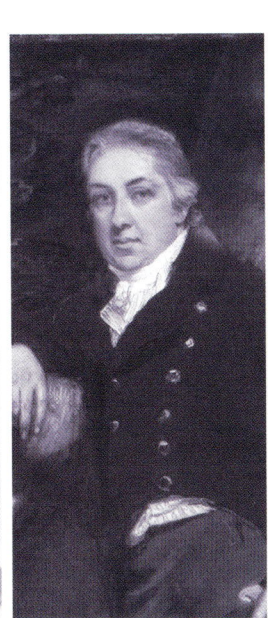

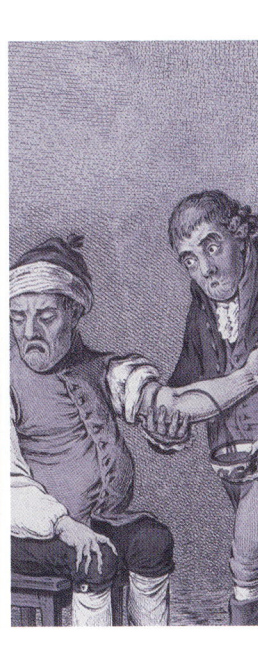

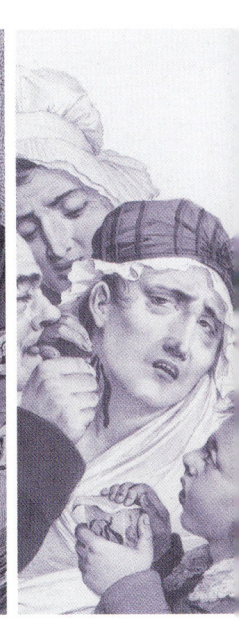

People have always searched for remedies for illnesses in order to live healthier and longer lives. Some of these remedies have changed over time, but others have remained the same for many centuries.

THE USE OF TRADITIONAL TREATMENTS AND REMEDIES

Herbal medicines

There is evidence worldwide that farming societies used herbs and plants before modern medicines were available. In Britain, traces of herbs and plants have been found at prehistoric sites. Many of these are known to have been used later in various remedies, including chickweed, which was used to treat open sores or as an ointment for skin conditions, and violets, which have been used as an antiseptic and as a basis for cough medicines.

Herbs were used as ingredients in all medieval medicines. They were available to everyone, whether rich or poor. Some remedies would contain expensive ingredients imported from the Far East, whilst others would be made of herbs found in local fields and hedges. It is possible that, although some of these remedies may have worked, others may not have had any healing powers whatsoever. Poor people turned to the local wise woman for cures. Although these wise women may have been very skilled herbalists, they would not have been able to write and so there are no records of the medicines that they prepared.

Richer people consulted doctors, who followed recipes in books called 'herbals' to prepare their medicines. Although at one time historians considered these herbals almost useless, recent research has changed their opinions. The *Leech Book* of Bald, a ninth century Anglo-Saxon physician, contained hundreds of recipes for herbal remedies, along with sensible advice that had, in fact, been collected from ancient medicine. For example:

> "Work an eye salve for a wen [stye], take cropleek and garlic, of both equal quantities, pound them well together, take wine and bullocks gall, of both equal quantities, mix with the leek, put *this* then into a brazen vessel, let it stand nine days in the

35

well, put it into a horn, and about night time apply it with a feather to the eye: the best leechdom [medical remedy]."

From 'Leech Book. Book I (ii)', p.35 in Leechdoms, Wortcunning and Starcraft of Early England. *Collected and edited by the Rev. Oswald Cockayne, M.A. Cantab. Vol.II, 1865*

In the parish of Myddfai, in Carmarthenshire in west Wales, the legend of The Lady of the Lake is still remembered. According to the legend, a mysterious lady is said to have risen up from the lake called Llyn-y-Fan-Fach to seek out her eldest son, Rhiwallon Feddyg (Rhiwallon the Doctor). She then taught him how to ease pain and suffering through the medicinal properties of local plants and herbs. She foretold that Rhiwallon's sons would be the most skilled physicians in the country.

The Lady of the Lake may have been a legend, but the Physicians of Myddfai seem to be based on fact. Rhiwallon and his three sons, Cadwgan, Gruffudd and Einion, were court doctors to the Lord of Dinefwr during the thirteenth century. They wrote down their cures and remedies in order to share them with others. These can be found today in *Llyfr Coch Hergest (The Red Book of Hergest)*, which is kept at the Bodleian Library in Oxford.

SOURCE 1

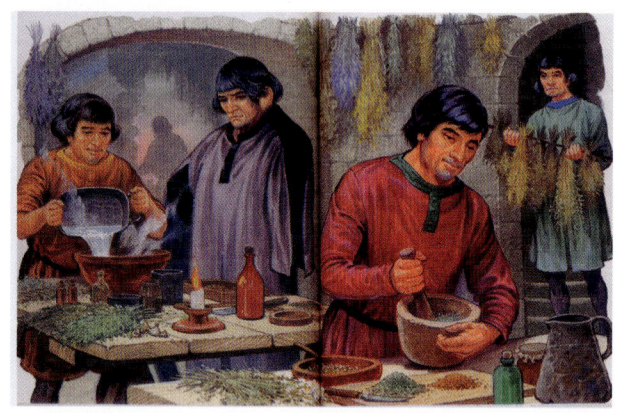

An artist's impression of the Physicians of Myddfai

Many of the physicians' medicines were made from herbs and plants collected from the fileds and hedgerows around Myddfai. They would grind the herbs using a **pestle and mortar**, then add boiling water to make herbal drinks, or mix them with plant oil to make ointments.

In order to treat a swelling in the spine doctors would use a mixture made by grinding the root of the golden celandine flower and mixing it with fennel, garlic, vinegar and butter. This mixture would be placed on a cloth and then wrapped around the patient's neck. A cure for a rotting wound, when gangrene was eating away at the flesh, was as follows:

"Take a black toad which is only able to crawl and beat it with a stick until it becomes angry and so that it swells until it dies. Then take it and put it in an earthenware cooking pot and close the lid on it so that the smoke cannot escape nor the air get into it. Burn the toad in the pot until it is ashes and put the ashes on the gangrene."

A paraphrse of a remedy by the Physicians of Myddfai from the Red Book of Hergest

Rhiwallon and his sons also followed the medieval tradition of studying the stars to help them find cures for their patients. They claimed that the movement of the planets told them what they should eat and drink every month of the year. In August, for example, they advised their patients to eat plenty of broth (*cawl*) and vegetables, and to put white pepper in their broth. They should also avoid drinking beer or mead (a sweet honey wine) during August.

These early doctors were also interested in preventing people from becoming ill. They advised bathing in cold water in the summer and then dressing in clean clothes. They also advised people to clean their teeth with the bark of dry hazel twigs, saying that these things would make them feel – and smell – better. This was the 'healthy living' advice of the time.

The Physicians of Myddfai may have learnt their ideas from traditions that had been passed down through many generation. They may also have learnt from other doctors in Europe at this time, who would have been using the same kind of medicines, and were experimenting with herbs and watching the stars.

Throughout the Middle Ages most illnesses were treated with herbal potions. They were not only used by doctors, but also by wise women and men (or healers) in villages and towns around the country. These healers possessed a great deal of knowledge about the use of herbs to treat everyday illnesses. Many locally grown plants were used and some medieval remedies were useful. Plantain was a very common ingredient. It was recommended for boils in the ear, dog bites, cuts and wounds. Modern analysis has shown that plantain is an antibiotic and in many remedies would have stopped infection.

Foreign herbs became increasingly popular as European voyagers sailed further and further to the Spice Islands in the Far East. After Columbus' voyage of discovery to America in 1492 (see Chapter 2) sugar was imported in large quantities. It was regarded as being very effective in the treatment of disease.

With the coming of the sixteenth century, we enter the period now known as the 'Medical Renaissance'. The invention of the printing press made it possible to produce many books, including 'herbals'. William Turner (c.1510-1568) was an English clergyman, physician and naturalist who has become known as 'the father of British botany'. He studied medicine and botany in Italy after leaving England to escape religious persecution during the Reformation era. He was the author of the first English works on plants: *Names of Herbs* (1548) and *A New Herball* (1551).

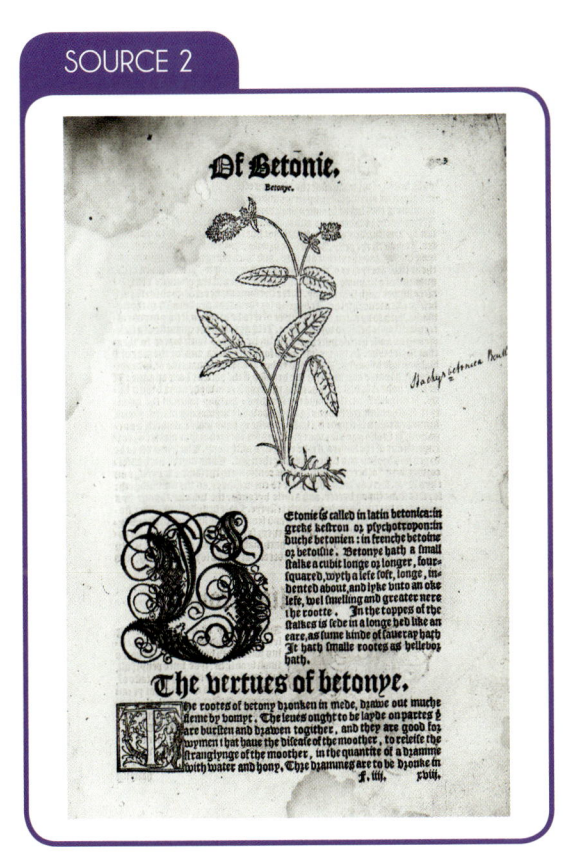

SOURCE 2

A page from Turner's A New Herball, *1551*

On the page shown in Source 2, Turner describes the benefits of the plant called betony: "The roots of betony drunk in mead draw out much phlegm by vomit." (The rootes of betony dronken in mede, drawe out muche fleme by vomyt.) Betony is a perennial plant that grows in grassland and open woods. It is still common in Wales and England. Turner also named many other plants in his book, including goatsbeard and hawkweed.

Another prominent character in this Medical Renaissance period was Lady Grace Mildmay (1552-1620), also previously referred to in Chapter 2. Lady Grace was born into a wealthy family and typically for the time she was expected to provide medical care for the people who lived on her family's lands. Medicinal knowledge was therefore part of her education.

When Lady Grace was a young girl, her governess had made her read Turner's *A New Herball*. It was here that she first found out about herbs and their medicinal uses. She had a thirst for knowledge and read widely in order to increase her medical understanding. She discussed medical matters with doctors and wrote down many of her treatments.

Lady Grace's favourite medicine, which she called her 'precious balm', took five weeks to make and involved fifteen separate processes. Herbs and seeds made up the majority of the ingredients in all of her treatments but there were also items that were new to Europe, like tobacco. Occasionally her treatments also included things like elk's hooves, crabs' claws and powder of human skull.

With her collection of medicines, Lady Grace tackled a wide range of illnesses, including jaundice, smallpox, skin diseases, cramp, ulcers, loss of memory, fevers of all kinds, eye problems and **melancholy**.

SOURCE 3

Take diascordium 1 ounce; mithridate 2 ounces; syrup of lemons 1 ounce. Mix these with cardus benedictus water or angelica water ¼ of a pint. Take 3 pints of small ale; three handfuls of sorrel; 2 handfuls of the tops of marigolds. Steep them in the ale all night and in the morning strain it out hard and make some posset drink of it. And every 4 hours take a spoonful of the cordial water above written, in a draught of this posset ale. ...
(I give this cordial in this manner. Some times but once a day for 3 days together, that is at 9 of the clock at night. And all the mornings after give every hour to drink a draught of broth warm, made with the strength of a good chicken, a crust of bread, a whole mace, endive, borage, violet leaves, cinquefoil, strawberry leaves, of each a like [amount], in all a pretty bundle

Lady Grace Mildmay's recommended treatment for a burning fever

Up until the mid eighteenth century, preparing medicines continued to be part of upper-class women's everyday work and many women of this class, like Lady Grace, wrote books containing recipes for remedies for fevers, coughs, stomach pains and even for smallpox. These medicines were made from herbs grown in their gardens. *Elinor Fettiplace's Receipt Book* (1604) contained many remedies for treating illnesses. For an extreme cough, the recipe suggested barley water flavoured with herbs, brown sugar candy, red rosewater and syrup of green ginger. *The Accomplish't Lady's Delight* (1675) included methods of making medicines and still recommended the use of herbs:

- For whooping cough: mixtures of dropwort and comfrey;
- For diarrhoea: rhubarb, aniseed, marshmallow root – a teaspoonful five or six times a day;
- For asthma: the bark of the cranberry bush, mixed with skullcap, skunk cabbage, cloves, capsicum, sherry. Take half a wineglass two or three times a day.

However, after 1750, few recipe books contained sections on medicine. The role of upper-class women was changing. It was no longer considered acceptable for them to do any work. There was also an increase in the number of doctors and, in the rapidly growing towns of the Industrial Revolution era, it was becoming impossible to grow the herbs needed for medicines.

TASKS

1. What does Source 1 show you about herbal medicines?
2. Why was William Turner important in the development of traditional treatments for disease?
3. Describe Lady Grace Mildmay's contribution to herbal medicines.

Barber surgeons

We have seen in Chapter 2 that Ambroise Paré was apprenticed to a barber surgeon. The medieval barber surgeons were some of the most common medical practitioners of the time. They would normally learn their trade as apprentices to more experienced colleagues and one of their main roles was to look after wounded soldiers during or after the numerous battles that occurred in the late Middle Ages.

Physicians, who had been trained at medical school, looked down on barber surgeons. Surgery was not studied because it was not considered a true part of medicine, so barber surgeons filled the gap, carrying out work such as bloodletting, extracting teeth, selling medicines, performing minor surgery and, of course, cutting hair. This is why today surgeons are addressed as 'Mister' and not 'Doctor'.

Surgery was not taught in most medical schools and the Christian church forbade dissection of human bodies for much of the Middle Ages. This meant that 'surgeons' tended to do the job part-time and treated only minor wounds. The frequent wars during the Middle Ages meant that some surgeons, like Paré, were able to gain experience on the battlefield. However, they would not have learnt very much as they had to work so quickly and in terrible conditions.

SOURCE 4

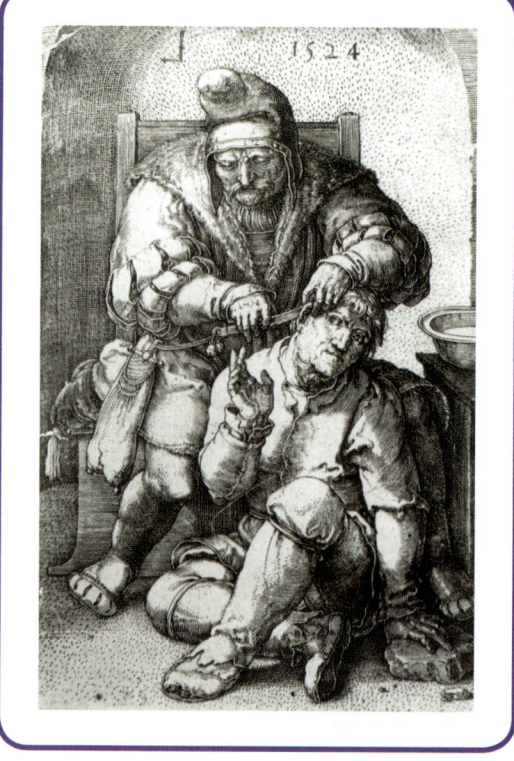

A barber surgeon in the sixteenth century, operating on a patient's head

Until the eighteenth century surgery was considered to be a trade rather than a profession. Barber surgeons used the same tools for many different jobs and they were not aware of the need to keep instruments clean. In any case, they would not have had clean running water on their premises at that time. They carried out their trade in a semi-public manner, in shops open to the street where anyone could watch. Signs outside these shops carried messages such as 'shaving, bleeding and teeth drawn with a touch'. They were also marked with a red and white pole representing bandages and blood. These poles can still be seen outside some barbers' shops today.

As well as making wigs, cutting hair and carrying out small operations the village barber also sold pills and ointments.

SOURCE 5

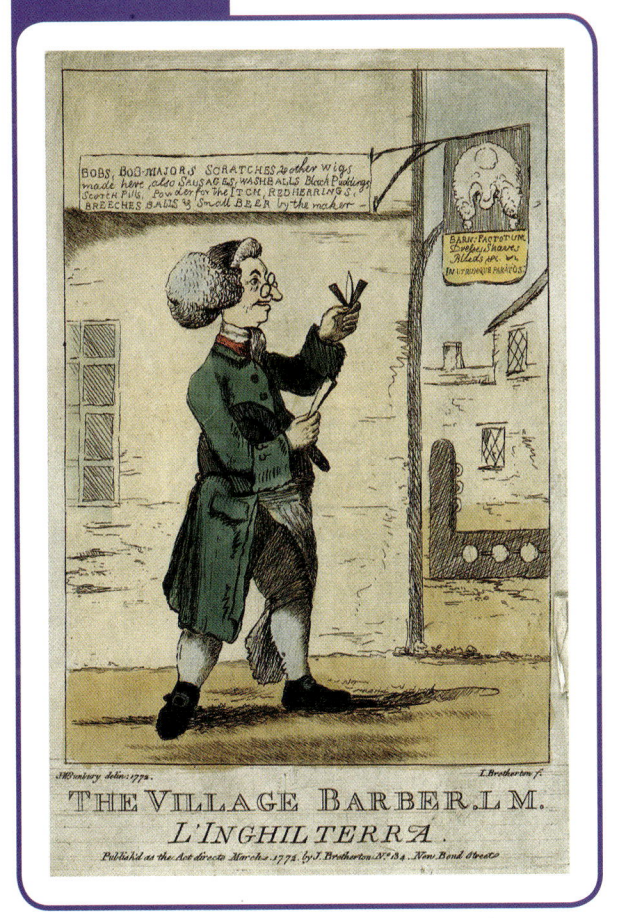

The eighteenth century village barber and pill seller

As barber surgeons were regarded as tradesmen, they operated within a trade guild system. In 1540 they had been granted a royal charter by King Henry VIII and had become 'The Company of Barber Surgeons'. However, in 1745 the surgeons split from the barbers. Surgery then became recognised as a profession, but barber surgeons continued to offer their trade to poorer people and still did a lot of bloodletting.

Purging, bloodletting and the use of leeches

Purging and bloodletting were both believed to be means of restoring the balance of the humours and purifying the body. Purging emptied the bowels and removed the poisons that had been held within the body. Like many others in the sixteenth century Lady Grace Mildmay still believed in the traditional theory of the four humours. She believed that imbalances in the human body led to illness. She suggested purges to empty the body of excess humours, but these purges should not be too extreme. Lady Grace stated in her written work:

> "It is [a] dangerous thing to wear and distract the humours in the body by extreme purges or extreme cordials. Whereby humours are stirred and made to fly up to the head, heart and spirits to the great molestation of all the said principal parts"

One method of purging involved pumping a liquid into the bowels through the rectum. A tube was used with a cleaned out pig's bladder attached, to act as a pump. The liquid 'purge' was made up of herbs, honey and water. After it had been given, the body would evacuate the purge in due course, releasing the poisons that had been held within the body.

Lady Grace also believed in bleeding her patients. Bloodletting meant draining varying amounts of blood from the body. Monastery records from the Middle Ages suggest that monks were bled between seven and twelve times a year and bloodletting was still very common well into the nineteenth century.

SOURCE 6

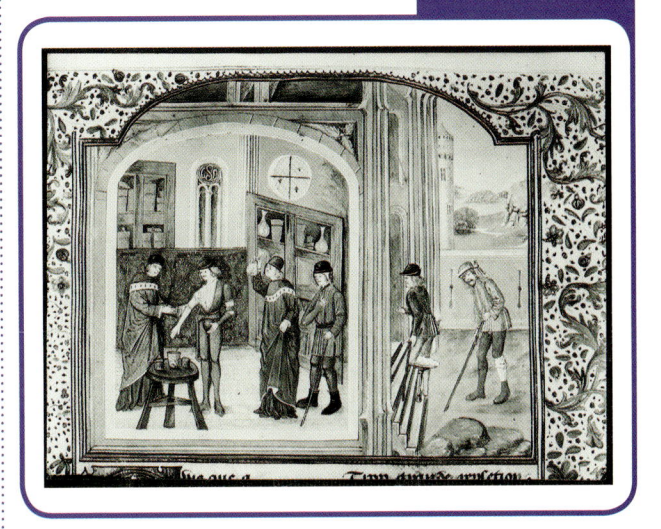

Bloodletting in medieval times

There were several techniques for bloodletting:
- When large amounts of blood needed to be drained a vein was cut and the blood was collected in a bowl;
- To release moderate amounts of blood, a bleeding cup could be used. This involved making a tiny cut on a patient's body and covering it with a heated cup, which remained in place by suction and drew out some of the patient's blood;
- To release small amounts of blood, blood-sucking leeches could be used.

Bloodletting was still one of the most common ways of treating many different illness in the sixteenth century. One of Lady Grace's cures for smallpox began:

"let the patient['s] blood, of the liver vein of the right arm, and that a reasonable quantity, according as you see the blood, good or corrupt, and according to the patient's age and strength."

According to a medical handbook of the time this procedure had many benefits, including: clearing the mind and improving memory, cleaning the guts and boosting digestion, enhancing hearing, making the patient less sleepy and anxious, cleaning the blood of poisons, producing clear urine and curing many pains and illnesses.

Given these wide-ranging benefits, it is not surprising that bloodletting was common. The bleeding sometimes continued until the patient was almost unconscious, by which time they may have lost three or four pints of blood.

Statistics have shown that, while bloodletting was of some use in treating some diseases when done in moderation and at the beginning of the disease, it had no effect in other diseases or at other times. However, many people still demanded bleeding or purging well into the nineteenth century, for all kinds of complaints, or even at the change of the seasons. This was the traditional way of doing things and, at that time, there was no way of curing or preventing diseases.

SOURCE 7

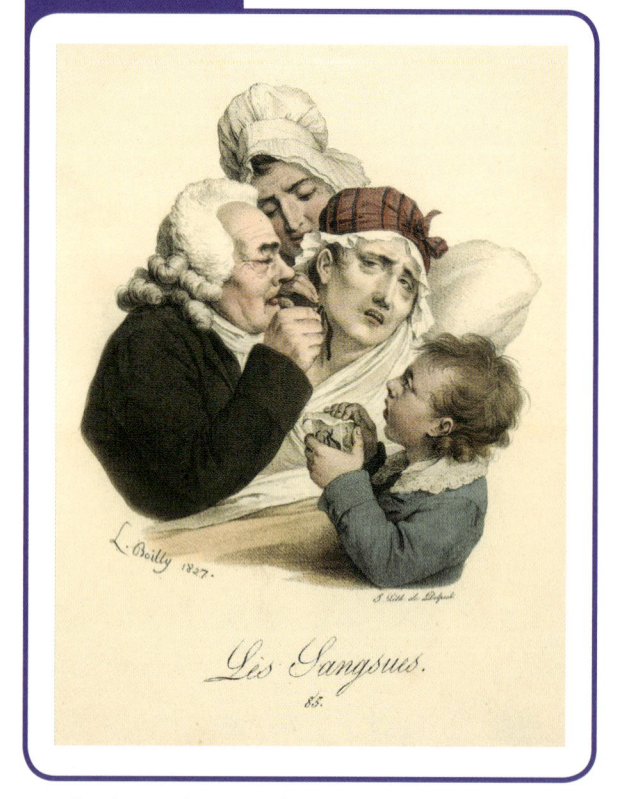

An nineteenth century doctor applying leeches to bleed a patient

SOURCE 8

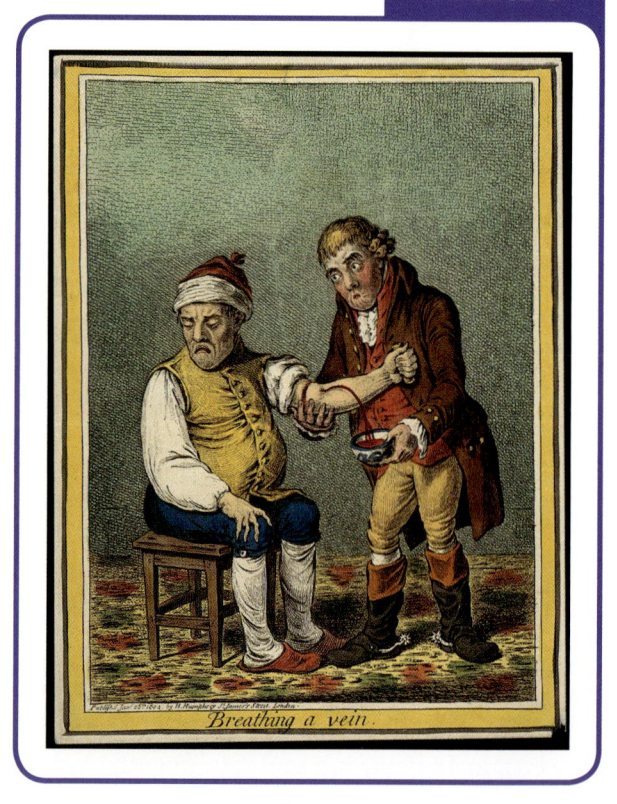

A doctor bleeding a patient from his arm, 1804

TASKS

1. Describe the work of barber surgeons.
2. Explain why purging was considered important for the human body.
3. Use the sources in this section and your own knowledge to explain the different methods of bloodletting.

SCIENTIFIC APPROACHES TO TREATING DISEASE

Ancient ideas about medicine had dominated in Europe for more than 1500 years. However, during the Renaissance of the sixteenth and seventeenth centuries, a better understanding of anatomy and advances in scientific knowledge had begun to challenge these long-held ideas.

In the eighteenth century, modern science began to develop. Instead of looking for ideas in translations of ancient medical books, scientists now adopted the recommendations of Paracelsus and others to use their own detailed observation, experiment and measurements to build up an accurate picture of the natural world. During this 'scientific revolution' old explanations that had served the western world so well and for so long – like those of Galen – were questioned and, if they were found to be inaccurate, abandoned.

Gradually the works of the ancient writers became less and less important. New treatments and ideas about disease developed to replace the old. These new ideas developed at different times and at different speeds, but some of the old treatments continued to be used because there were no alternatives.

The invention of the microscope

The Renaissance had inspired many new inventions across Europe, and some of these helped in the advancement of medical knowledge. In 1609 the Dutch spectacle-maker Janssen used two lenses to make a simple microscope. The Italian physician Sanctorius had developed the thermometer by 1630; this was an important aid in diagnosing illness. Malpighi (1628-94), an Italian anatomist, invented a more efficient microscope that could be used to study blood. He used this microscope to confirm that Harvey's ideas were correct, as he was able to see the minute blood vessels (capillaries) that link the arteries with the veins.

In 1661 King Charles II of England founded the Royal Society. Its aim was to use experiments to advance knowledge. The Royal Society tried to encourage a scientific approach to looking at things and this way of thinking helped to develop an understanding of disease. Englishman Robert Hooke (1635-1703) was a member of the Royal Society and he improved on the early microscopes.

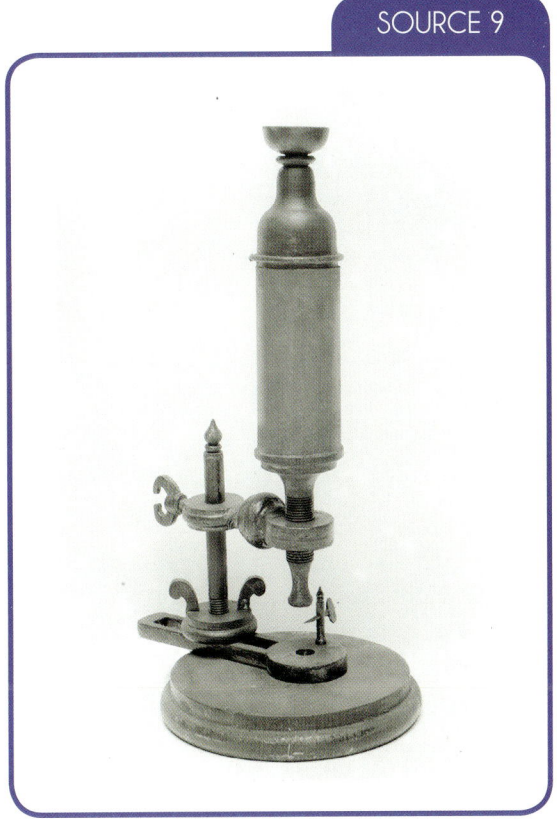

SOURCE 9

A model of Robert Hooke's microscope

Dutch clockmaker Anton van Leeuwenhoek also made some improvements to the early microscopes. Although the images provided by Leeuwenhoek's simple single-lens microscope were fuzzy, he found that everything that he studied through his lens contained tiny organisms. He discovered these tiny organisms in food, drops of water, human excreta, animal intestines and even in the material that he scraped from between his own teeth. He published his findings in a series of papers for the Royal Society in London.

As scientists had started to examine the link between germs and disease, Leeuwenhoek's discovery of the tiny organisms interested other scientists, but microscopes in the seventeenth and eighteenth centuries were not good enough to study any further. However, by the early nineteenth century, purer and clearer glass was being produced and in 1830 Joseph Lister, a British scientist and father of the later Lord Joseph Lister, developed a much stronger microscope. This could magnify 1,000 times without distortion. Scientists were now able to examine micro-organisms in greater detail. A much more scientific approach to studying disease was now possible.

SOURCE 10

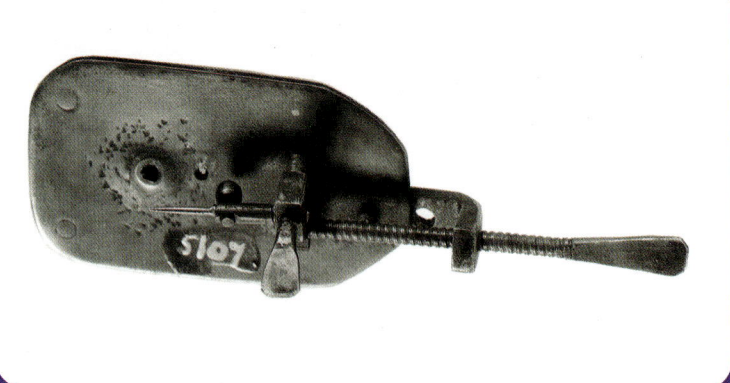

An exact copy of the Leeuwenhoek microscope

Scientific study of disease

New medical schools were opened and old ones were transformed. The new ideas and techniques that were being developed were spread through better training for doctors. It became part of a doctor's training to carry out dissections, to use microscopes and to think scientifically. By the eighteenth century, it was getting increasingly hard to get bodies on which trainee doctors could practise in their anatomy classes. Some bodies were snatched from graveyards and, later in the century, hospitals asked the workhouses for the bodies of dead paupers.

As scientific study of disease increased, the medical books of the ancient writers were discarded and the Catholic Church, often an obstacle to new methods of treating disease, was no longer in control of medical training.

Scientists gradually discovered that many ancient ideas about the natural world, especially the theory of the four elements that had formed the basis of the theory of the four humours, were wrong. They discovered that air itself is made up of different gases. Irish-born Robert Boyle (1627-91) worked as an assistant to Robert Hooke in the 1650s. He devoted himself to the study of gases and carried out experiments on air, combustion and respiration.

New medicines were also discovered, including digitalis, which was developed by the English physician William Withering (1741-99), who published his *Account of the Foxglove* in 1785. He had obtained a traditional remedy for dropsy (the accumulation of fluid in the human body, which is one symptom of heart failure) from a woman in his native Shropshire. Withering believed that one of the herbal ingredients in the remedy was responsible for curing dropsy. He tried each individual ingredient out on animals and then on patients. He finally discovered that foxglove (*digitalis purpurea*) was the effective ingredient. As a result of his discovery, digitalis was used as a drug for heart disease.

Withering had used scientific methods to study a traditional remedy and had discovered which component was responsible for curing the illness. This technique was later used to find treatments for the dreaded disease of smallpox.

TASKS

1. Explain why there was a 'scientific revolution' in the eighteenth century.
2. Describe the benefits that the invention of the microscope brought to the study of disease.
3. How successful was the work of William Withering in the treatment of disease?
4. Create a timeline from the section above to show how developments in science helped in the study of disease.

Edward Jenner and vaccination

Smallpox was a disease that terrified people in the eighteenth century. Epidemics of smallpox had been sweeping through Europe since the sixteenth century. It affected rich and poor alike and there was no cure. The death rate was high. Those who survived were often left deaf, blind, brain damaged or physically disabled. Its marks did not go away and people's faces and bodies were often badly disfigured with pockmarks left behind by the disease.

SOURCE 11

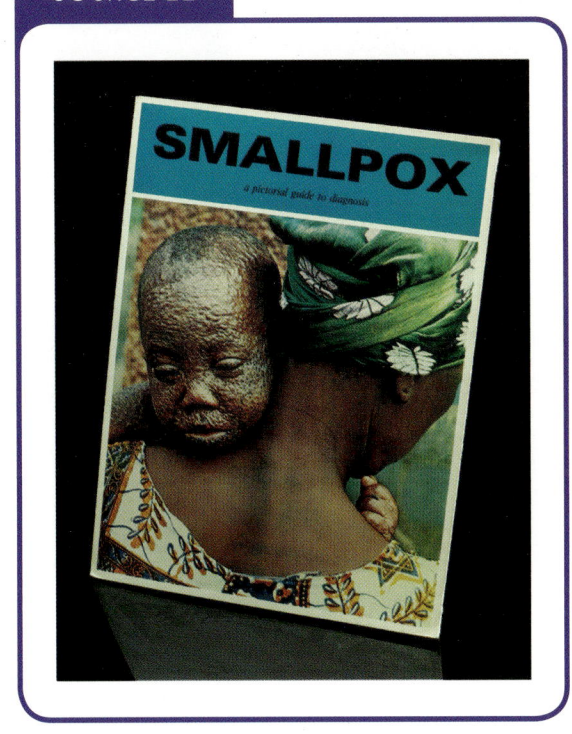

A photograph of a 20th century victim of smallpox

Epidemics of smallpox broke out in Britain every few years. The virus was spread from person to person through coughs and sneezes and through touch. The scientific approach to treating disease in the eighteenth century focused strongly on trying to prevent smallpox. Two methods were developed: **inoculation** and **vaccination**.

Inoculation

One method of preventing smallpox was discovered in China. Doctors there had noticed that people who had suffered a mild form of smallpox often survived when there were later epidemics of the disease. They developed a method called inoculation, which involved spreading matter from a smallpox scab onto an open cut in the skin. This gave people a mild dose and protected them from the full effects of a future attack.

This method of inoculation spread along the trade routes from China through Asia and to Turkey, where it was observed by Lady Mary Wortley Montagu (1689-1762).

Whilst living in Constantinople (Istanbul) where her husband was Ambassador, Lady Mary had seen Turkish women inoculating children. In a letter that she wrote in 1717 she commented:

> "The small pox, so fatal, and so general amongst us, is here entirely harmless, by the invention of *engrafting*, grafting, which is the term they give to it. There is a set of old women, who make it their business to perform the operation, every autumn, in the month of September, when the great heat is abated. … There is no example of any one that has died in it, and you may believe I am well satisfied of the safety of this experiment, since I intend to try it on my dear little son."

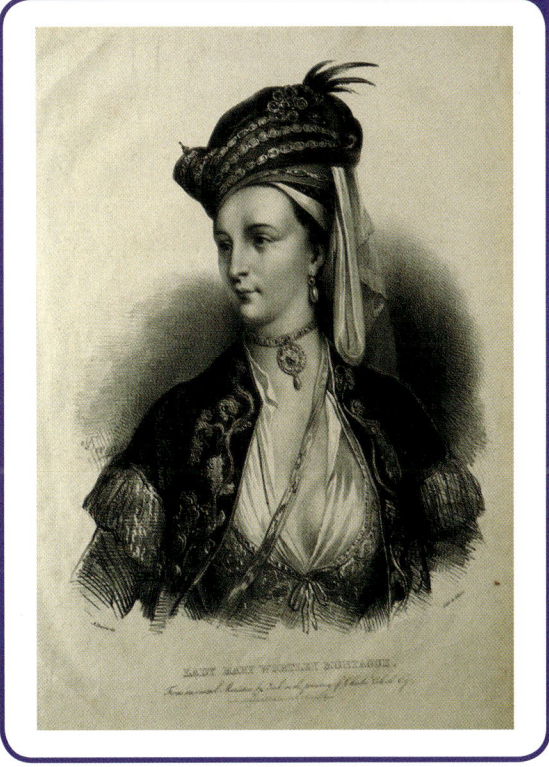

SOURCE 12

Lady Mary Wortley Montagu

Lady Mary herself had survived an attack of smallpox two years earlier and did not want her children to suffer from the same disfiguring disease. In 1717 she had her three-year old son inoculated. In 1721, after her return to England, there was a severe smallpox epidemic that caused 3,000 deaths in London. She insisted that her English doctors inoculated her three-year old daughter. Both of her children survived the smallpox epidemic.

Many of Lady Mary's friends were doctors, and as she was a very influential person she was able to persuade them to make use of inoculation. Even the royal family was impressed by this new method. King George I (1714-1727) gave physicians permission to try out inoculation on six prisoners in Newgate Jail and on eleven pauper children. The trials were successful and it soon became fashionable for the upper class to have their children inoculated. Doctors saw the potential – and the profit – in smallpox inoculation, for which they charged a fee. It soon became big business whenever smallpox epidemics raged in Britain in the eighteenth century. Inoculation became common and some doctors became rich through mass inoculation.

During an epidemic in Kent in 1766, surgeons Robert Sutton and his son Daniel, carried out mass inoculations. It was recorded that:

> "the Suttons, father and son … in eleven years inoculated 2,514 people, for substantial fees. They also sold, for anything between fifty and a hundred pounds, to practitioners living at a safe distance from them, the secrets of their special method … They had their own inoculation house … where patients were prepared for the operation and rested after it."

From Doctor Jenner of Berkeley, *Dorothy Fisk*, 1959

James Woodforde (1740-1803) was a parson and a diarist. He recorded in his diary:

> **November 3rd 1776:** This morning about 11 o'clock Dr Thorne … came to my House and inoculated my two servants … Pray God my People and all others in the Small Pox may do well, several Houses have got the Small Pox at present in Weston. O Lord send thy Blessing of Health on them all.
> **November 22nd 1776:** John Bowles's Wife is under Inoculation … My neighbour Downing, the Father of the Children that were lately inoculated has got the small pox in the natural way and likely to have it very bad … I sent over Harry Dunnell this evening to Dr Thorne's, to desire him to come to-morrow and see him, which he promised.

Diary of a Country Parson: The Reverend James Woodforde, 1758-1891, edited by John Beresford, 1924, pp. 190, 192

Inoculation undoubtedly reduced the likelihood of dying from smallpox, but it was by no means safe. Some people died of the mild dose that they were given. Others became carriers of the disease and could spread it to people with whom they came into contact. A more effective and safer way of preventing smallpox was needed.

Vaccination

In the late 1790s Edward Jenner (1749-1823), who worked as a doctor at Chipping Sodbury in Gloucestershire, used a traditional remedy to develop a safer method of preventing the smallpox disease.

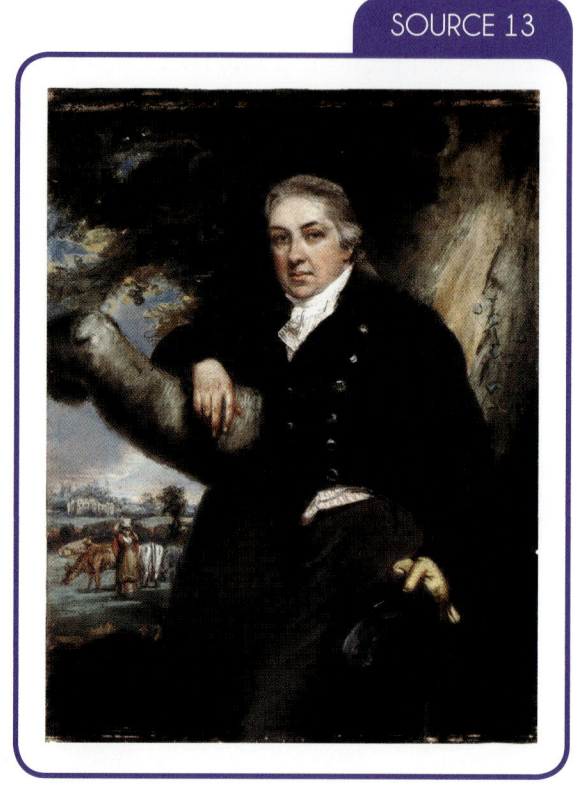

SOURCE 13

Edward Jenner

A dairymaid once told him that she would not catch smallpox because she had already had cowpox, which was a mild illness. Jenner decided to test this theory. In 1798 he wrote:

> "it commonly happens that a disease is communicated to the cows, and from the cows to the dairymaids … Inflamed spots … begin to appear on different parts of the hands … and sometimes on the wrists …
>
> what renders the cow-pox virus so extremely singular [unusual] is that the person who has been thus affected is forever after secure from the infection of the smallpox …
>
> The more accurately to observe the progress of the infection I selected a healthy boy, about eight years old, for the purpose of inoculation for the cow-pox. The matter was taken from a sore on the hand of a dairymaid [Sarah Nelmes], who was infected by her master's cows, and it was inserted, on the 14th of May, 1796, into the arm of the boy by means of two superficial incisions …"

On the seventh day he complained of uneasiness in the axilla [armpit], and on the ninth he became a little chilly, lost his appetite, and had a slight headache. … but on the day following he was perfectly well. …

In order to ascertain whether the boy … was secure from the contagion of the smallpox, he was inoculated … with variolous [smallpox] matter … but no disease followed. … Several months afterwards he was again inoculated with variolous matter, but no sensible effect was produced on the constitution."

From On Vaccination Against Smallpox, *Edward Jenner, Dodo Press, 2009, pp. 1, 2, 3, 12, 13*

Jenner tried the same experiment on a number of other people. Only then did he conclude "that the cow-pox protects the human constitution from the infection of the smallpox". He had discovered a treatment for smallpox that has become known as 'vaccination' (so called after the Latin word for a cow, vacca). Jenner wrote up his findings and submitted them to the Royal Society for publication in 1798. However, there was a great deal of opposition to Jenner's ideas and the Royal Society rejected his work.

SOURCE 14

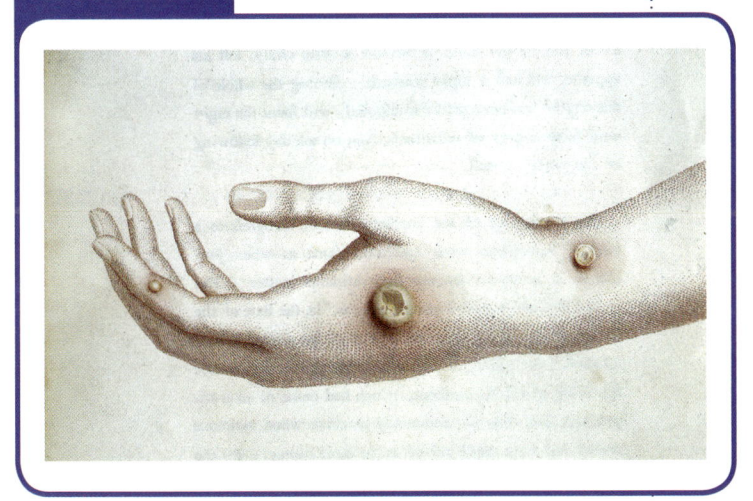

Cowpox scabs on Sarah Nelmes' hand

Jenner therefore published his findings himself. He called his work *An Inquiry into the Causes and Effects of the Variolae Vaccinae, A Disease Discovered in Some of the Western Counties of England, Particularly Gloucestershire, and Known by the Name of the Cow Pox* (1798). His book was widely read and parliament thought that Jenner's work was very important: in 1802 he was given a grant of £30,000 to open a vaccination clinic in London.

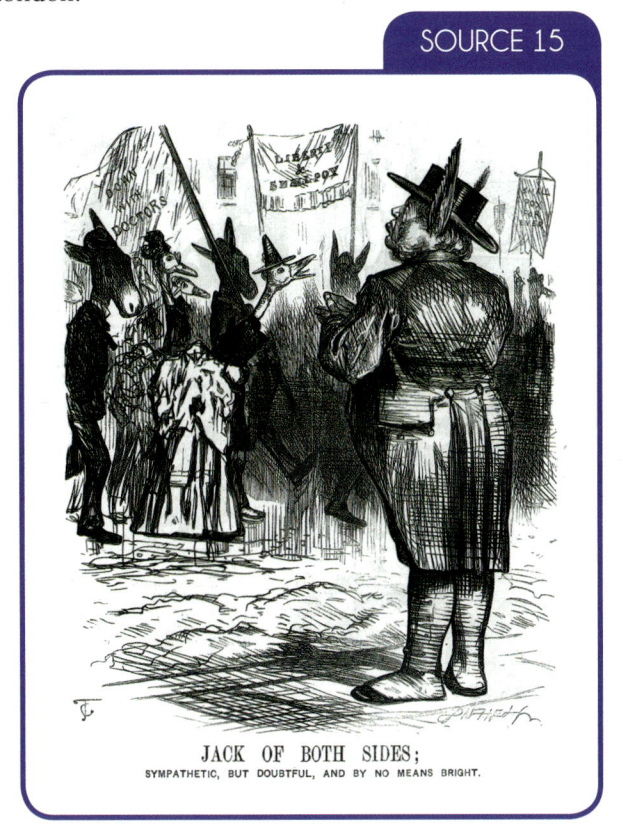

SOURCE 15

JACK OF BOTH SIDES;
SYMPATHETIC, BUT DOUBTFUL, AND BY NO MEANS BRIGHT.

A cartoon showing what some people thought might happen if humans were inoculated with cowpox

By 1803 doctors were using the vaccination technique in America. In 1805 the French Emperor Napoleon had all his soldiers vaccinated and by 1812 translations of Jenner's work were being sold in central Asia. In 1852, more than 50 years after Jenner's discovery, the British government made vaccination compulsory.

Chance, scientific investigation and government action had all been important in the discovery and development of vaccination. Even so, there continued to be opposition to the procedure.

- Some people opposed vaccination simply because it was new;
- Some could not believe that a disease that came from cows could protect people from a human disease like smallpox;
- Doctors who were making money out of inoculations did not want to lose that income;
- Vaccination was seen as dangerous. Some patients died when some careless doctors infected them

SOURCE 16

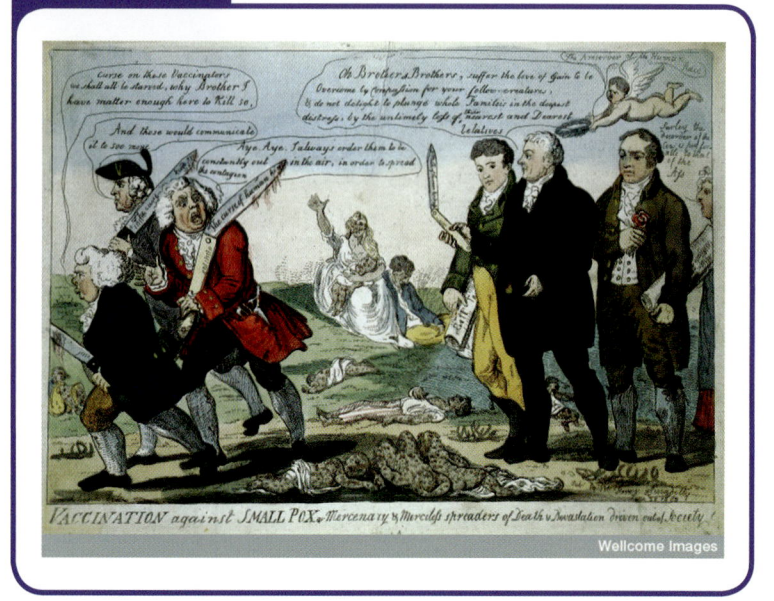

An anti-vaccination cartoon, 1808

with smallpox instead of cowpox; and some doctors used infected needles, that led to the death of their patients;
- Vaccination was not free. The system was unfair. The poor could not afford vaccination;
- Making vaccination compulsory was regarded as an attack on personal liberty;
- Herbalists opposed vaccination because it meant less work for them.

Jenner's work was an important turning point and he is regarded as the first immuniser. Although he did not realise it at the time, vaccination worked because cowpox is a similar virus to smallpox – when the human body reacts to cowpox it also becomes immune to other similar diseases. Vaccination against smallpox has become compulsory in most countries and since 1977 there have been no recorded cases of the disease. In 1979 the World Health Organization declared smallpox extinct.

SOURCE 17

Jenner was the first immuniser. He made deliberate use of the knowledge that recovering from a mild form of a disease gives human beings protection (or immunity) against a more severe form. This was the basis of the science of immunology which was to be pursued with such success by Pasteur and others half a century later.

Historians I. Dawson and I. Coulson, writing in Medicine and Health through time, *2000*

TASKS

1. What is inoculation?
2. How important was Lady Mary Wortley Montagu in the fight against smallpox?
3. What is vaccination? Explain why there was opposition to Jenner's discovery of vaccination.
4. What has been the long-lasting effect of Jenner's discovery?

Examination practice

This section provides guidance on how to answer Question 1(d), 2(d) and 3(d) from Unit 3. The question is worth 8 marks.

Question 1(d), 2(d), 3(d) – the selection of own knowledge and the analysis of key concepts

Why was the use of vaccination by Edward Jenner in the late eighteenth century a turning point in the prevention and treatment of disease?

[8 marks]

Tips on how to answer

- The reference to turning point in the question **implies a sharp change in direction of treatment**;
- The thrust of the question **is about change** and **the causes of that change**;
- You need to consider what came **before** the event mentioned in the question and compare this with what came **afterwards**, noting **the change and the reasons for that change**;
- You need to support your observations with **specific factual detail**;
- Remember that this question requires you to **provide a judgement**, giving specific reasons why you think the event was a turning point.

Response by candidate one

Edward Jenner was a doctor in Gloucestershire. He injected matter from a cowpox sore on the hand of a dairymaid called Sarah Nelmes into the arm of an 8-year-old boy. The boy became ill with cowpox but when he was later inoculated with smallpox, he did not get the disease. Jenner had found a method of preventing people from getting the killer disease of smallpox.

Examiner's comment

The candidate provides an answer that is descriptive rather than analytical and evaluative. There is no reference to turning point and reference to change is only implied. This is a limited answer, which only meets the requirements of Level One. It is worth 3 marks.

Response by candidate two

Epidemics of the killer disease smallpox had broken out in Britain every few years from the sixteenth century. Smallpox affected rich and poor alike. The death rate was high and there was no cure for it. Even if a victim survived, they could be left severely disabled and disfigured.

A method of preventing smallpox had been discovered in China. It was called inoculation. This involved spreading matter from a smallpox scab onto an open cut in the skin. This gave people a mild dose of the smallpox disease and prevented a full attack of the disease. Inoculation was brought to Britain in the early eighteenth century when Lady Mary Montagu had her children inoculated. They survived a smallpox epidemic in 1721 but inoculation was not a safe method. Some people died of the small dose that they were given and others became carriers of the disease. A more effective and safer way of preventing smallpox was needed.

A Gloucestershire doctor, Edward Jenner, discovered a safer method at the end of the eighteenth century. His method was called vaccination. Cowpox was a similar disease to smallpox but much milder. Jenner injected matter from a cowpox sore on the hand of a dairymaid into an eight-year-old boy. The boy became ill with cowpox but, when he was later inoculated with smallpox, he did not develop the disease.

Jenner used scientific methods to prove that his use of vaccination protected people from smallpox. His discovery was a turning point in the prevention and treatment of disease because he published his findings in 1798 and made them available to a wide audience and because he had support from the government – he was given a grant of £30,000 in 1802 to open a vaccination clinic in London. This had not been done before. Jenner's use of vaccination was also a turning point because it led to the science of immunology and to the eventual eradication of a killer disease. In 1979 the World Health Organization declared that smallpox was extinct.

Examiner's comment

The candidate has produced a detailed answer, which is accurate and well informed. Observations are supported with specific factual detail. The candidate outlines the situation before Jenner's use of vaccination and then refers to Jenner's changes and what his discovery led to. The final paragraph focuses fully on 'turning point' and the candidate makes a valid final judgement. The answer meets the requirements of Level Three and is worthy of maximum (8) marks.

Now you have a go

Why was the invention of the microscope in the seventeenth century a turning point in the prevention and treatment of disease?

[8 marks]

CHAPTER 5

WHAT WERE THE MAIN ADVANCES MADE IN SURGICAL METHODS IN BRITAIN IN THE NINETEENTH CENTURY?

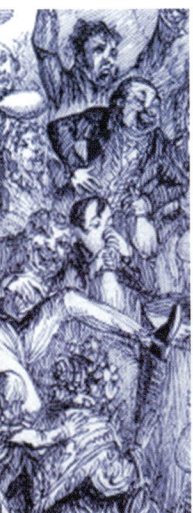

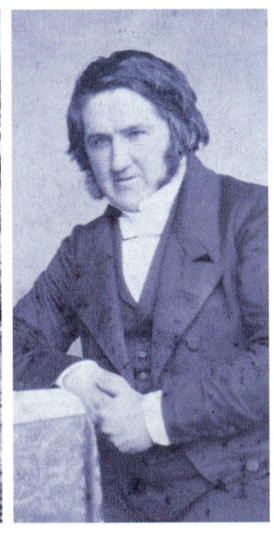

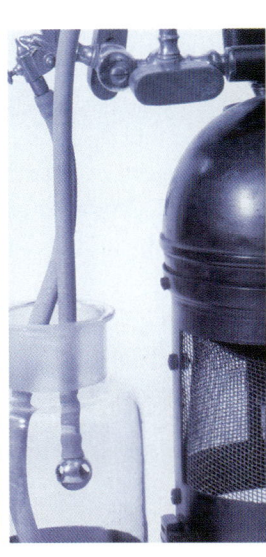

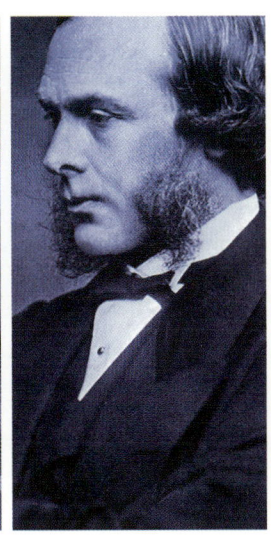

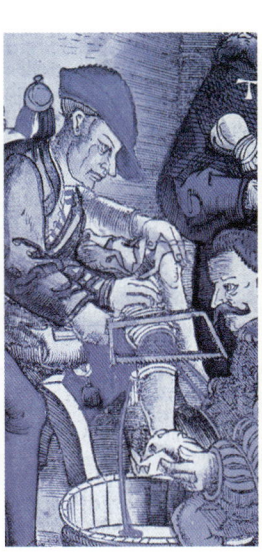

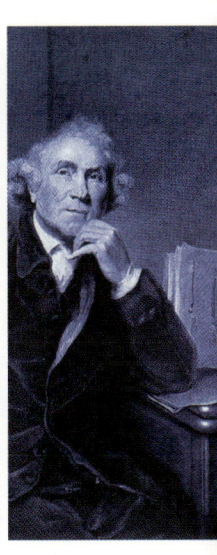

Before the eighteenth century most people who studied medicine did not study surgery because it was not thought to be a true part of medicine. It was not taught in the universities and the only way to become a surgeon was to be apprenticed to another surgeon and copy their work.

In the sixteenth century Ambroise Paré had been apprenticed to a barber surgeon and later became an army surgeon, learning as much as he could about treating wounds on the battlefield. He had discovered the use of ligatures to stop bleeding, but ligatures could carry infection and as yet there was nothing to stop infection nor to help patients deal with extreme pain.

During the seventeenth century surgery began to be taken more seriously. Richard Wiseman (1622-76) was surgeon to King Charles II from 1660. He had learned his skills through thirty years of work as a barber surgeon on the battlefield. In order to pass on his knowledge to younger surgeons he published two books: *A Treatise on Wounds* (1672) and *Several Surgical Treatises* (1676).

The books mostly described the cases that Wiseman had encountered on the battlefield and, although this was useful to younger barber surgeons, they offered very little that was new. So surgery carried on in the way it had done for centuries. Surgeons dealt with minor problems only: they either cut off infected body parts or removed kidney stones.

SOURCE 1

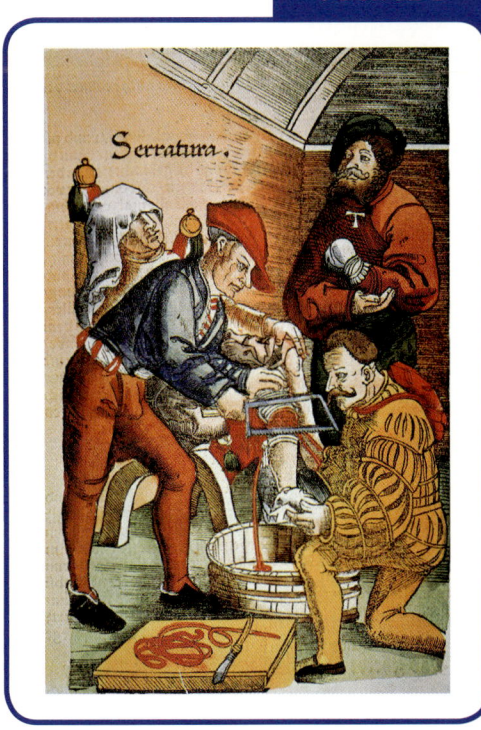

An amputation in the sixteenth century

All that they needed to perform an operation was a sharp knife, a strong saw and speed – a good surgeon took less than a minute to amputate an arm or a leg.

SOURCE 2

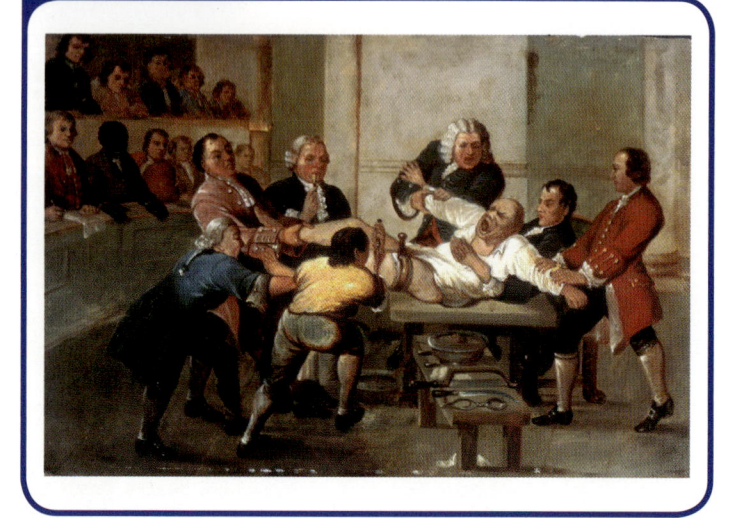

An operation c.1800

Source 1 shows a patient's bandaged leg being sawn through. The blood drips into a tub below the leg. There was no other way to operate at this time and the only comfort for the patient was to have a priest in attendance. In Source 2 the patient is held firmly and may have been told to bite hard on a piece of leather. Patients were sometimes blindfolded too. Although over a century apart, the method in both cases is very similar. The pain suffered must have been excruciating and the chance of infection was very high.

In the eighteenth century surgery started to be regarded as a part of medicine when surgeons, other than barber surgeons, began to practice in hospitals. The improving status of surgery was due to men like William Cheselden (1688-1752) who was a surgeon at St Thomas' Hospital in London. He became famous for carrying out successful operations. It is said that he could remove kidney stones in sixty seconds – the continued lack of anaesthetics meant that speed was all-important. Cheselden published *The Anatomy of the Human Body* in 1713 and later led a campaign for the recognition of surgery as a profession. In 1745 the Company of Surgeons was created, and this was to become the Royal College of Surgeons in 1800.

Although the status of surgery was improving, there were still serious problems to overcome in surgical procedures. Surgeons needed better training. The shortage of bodies on which to practise was a major problem. One option was to work with the bodies of executed criminals.

Another problem to be overcome was the lack of accommodation where surgeons could be trained.

In 1767 Scottish-born William Hunter (1718-83) set up a medical school at his house in Great Windmill Street in London, where he taught surgery. His brother John (1728-93), who had joined him in London as an assistant in 1748, trained there.

John Hunter has been referred to as a founder of 'scientific surgery'. He studied surgery under William Cheseldon and was to achieve even more fame than his elder brother. He worked as an assistant at St. Bartholomew's Hospital and later as a house surgeon at St George's Hospital. He was commissioned as an army surgeon in 1761 and served in France and Portugal for two years, where he had the opportunity to develop new ideas on how to treat war wounds. John Hunter also set up his own anatomy school, becoming a highly regarded teacher of anatomy and surgery. His famous pupils include Edward Jenner.

SOURCE 3

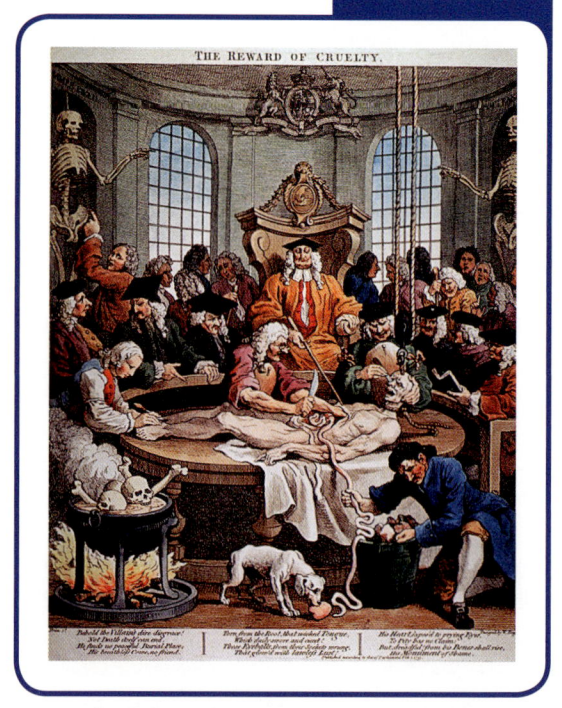

An eighteenth century print by William Hogarth, entitled The Reward of Cruelty, *showing an executed criminal being dissected in an anatomy class*

John Hunter wanted his contribution to surgery to be long lasting. In 1783 he moved to a large house in Leicester Square, where he established a teaching museum that housed his huge collection of plant and animal specimens. The house also contained his anatomy school, with teaching rooms and dissection facilities. The government purchased the Hunter Museum in 1799, and presented it to the Company of Surgeons, which later became the Royal College of Surgeons.

The efforts of the Hunter brothers had raised the status of surgery. The creation of the Royal College of Surgeons in London in 1800 meant that surgeons had to be registered and could therefore be taught properly, gaining proper qualifications. Modern surgery had begun, but the techniques of surgery still needed to be improved.

SOURCE 4

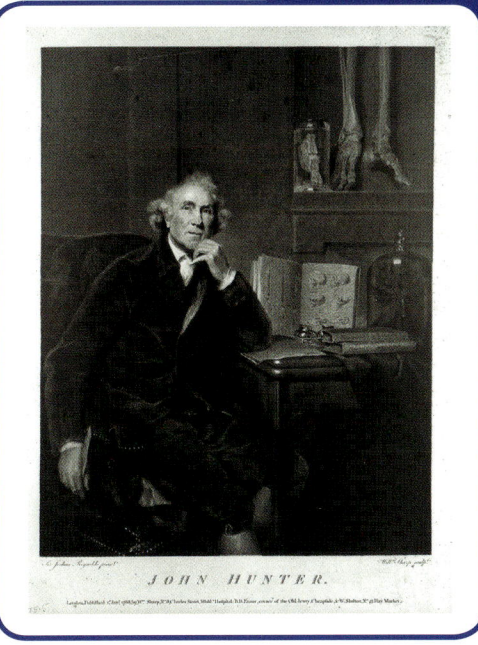

John Hunter

TASKS

1. Study Sources 1 and 2. What has changed and what has stayed the same in surgery?
2. How successful was William Cheselden as a surgeon?
3. What was John Hunter's contribution to surgery?

THE DEVELOPMENT OF ANAESTHETICS

Pain and infection were the two main problems in surgery. However, during the nineteenth century two major discoveries in particular improved surgical methods – anaesthetic and antiseptics.
- Anaesthetic was a substance, often a gas such as ether or chloroform, that produced unconsciousness before and during surgery. It helped to deal with pain.
- Antiseptics were chemicals that were used to destroy bacteria and prevent infection in a wound or cut.

The need for anaesthetic

Surgery in the early nineteenth century was still a dangerous and painful process. There was no way of completely relieving pain. Without anaesthetic, patients would be in unimaginable agony. Sometimes they were hypnotised into unconsciousness beforehand or, more likely, given enough alcohol to send them into a drunken stupor. Very often the pain suffered during an operation could lead to heart failure and death.

In order to limit the duration of pain, operations were carried out with as much speed as possible, but this could lead to drastic mistakes. Scottish-born Robert Liston (1794-1867) was professor of clinical surgery at University College, London. He once amputated a leg in two and a half minutes but worked so fast that he cut off his patient's testicles as well. During another high-speed amputation Liston cut off the fingers of his assistant and slashed the coat of a spectator who, believing that he had been stabbed, died of shock. Even worse was to follow as both the assistant and the patient died of infection.

Robert Liston became famous throughout Europe for his surgical skill. He published two very important books that helped to develop surgery: *Practical Surgery* (1837) and *Elements of Surgery* (1840).

However, there were a few operations that surgeons could carry out with some success:
- Amputating limbs;
- Trephining/trepanning (cutting a hole in the skull);
- Removing superficial tumours.

These operations continued to be carried out as quickly as possible and surgeons had to get used to ignoring the reactions of their patients. However, some surgeons began to think that if patients could be safely made unconscious they would have more time to operate and to improve their techniques.

The science of chemistry was also developing at this time and experiments had shown that some chemicals had an effect on the human body. Sir Humphry Davy (1778-1829), an English chemist and inventor of the safety lamp (Davy Lamp) for miners, discovered in 1799 that nitrous oxide reduced the feeling of pain and he suggested that it might be used in surgical operations.

SOURCE 5

In 1799 Sir Humphry Davy discovered that if he breathed in nitrous oxide gas [laughing gas] it sometimes had strange effects. He said:
'In cutting one of the unlucky teeth called dentes fapientiae, I experienced an extensive inflammation of the gum, accompanied with great pain …
On the day when the inflammation was most troublesome, I breathed three large doses of nitrous oxide. The pain … diminished'
This led him on to a very important conclusion:
'As nitrous oxide … appears capable of destroying physical pain, it may probably be used … during surgical operations in which no great effusion of blood takes place.'

From Researches, Chemical and Philosophical; Chiefly Concerning Nitrous Oxide or Dephlogisticated Nitrous Air, and Its Respiration *by Humphry Davy, 1800, pp. 465, 556*

However, nitrous oxide, or laughing gas as it also became known, had an uncontrollable effect on anyone who breathed it in. When members of the public realised the effects of this gas, they even organized 'laughing gas parties'.

Even so, nitrous oxide was used in some operations in the early nineteenth century. However, surgeons sought to discover a more stable substance until finally Michael Faraday, a pupil of Sir Humphry Davy, found that the fumes from liquid ether could relieve pain.

Robert Liston was the first surgeon in Britain to use ether as a general anaesthetic when he carried out an operation in public at University College Hospital, London, in December 1846. This pointed the way to a future of pain-free surgery.

SOURCE 6

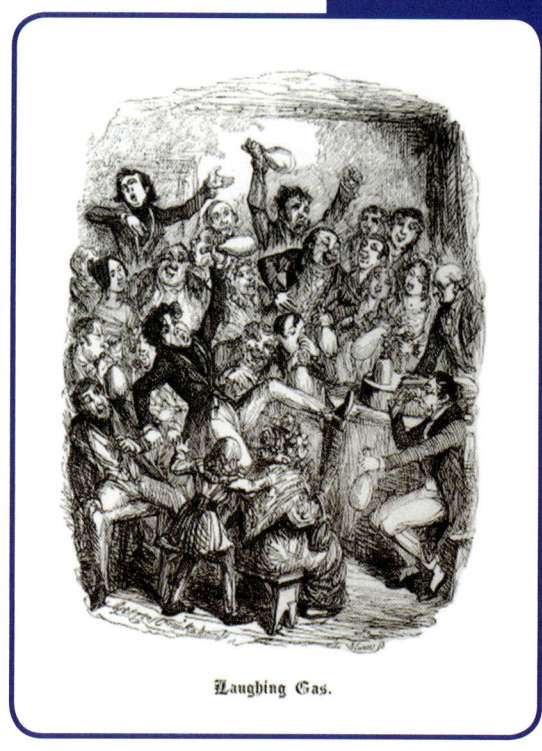

Laughing Gas.

A cartoon showing the audience at a lecture enjoying the effects of laughing gas, 1839

Unfortunately there were problems with using ether too. It irritated the lungs, causing the patient to cough during the operation. It was also unstable, had a nasty smell and produced inflammable vapour. A safer alternative was needed.

SOURCE 7

On 21 December 1846, Frederick Churchill, a thirty-six-year-old butler, was carried into the operating-theatre at University College Hospital, London, to have his left leg amputated. He was to become the most famous patient in surgical history. Churchill's operation was painless, for he was the first human being to have major surgery under an anaesthetic. …
Anaesthesia was the dawn of a new era in human welfare.

Historian William Armstrong, writing in an article entitled 'Under the Surgeon's knife' in History Makers: The Magazine that brings History to Life, *30 January 1970*

TASKS

1. Why were anaesthetics needed in surgery?
2. What was Robert Liston's contribution to surgery?
3. What were the advantages and disadvantages of using laughing gas in surgery?
4. Study Source 7. Why was the operation on Frederick Churchill a turning point in surgery?

James Simpson and the discovery of anaesthetics

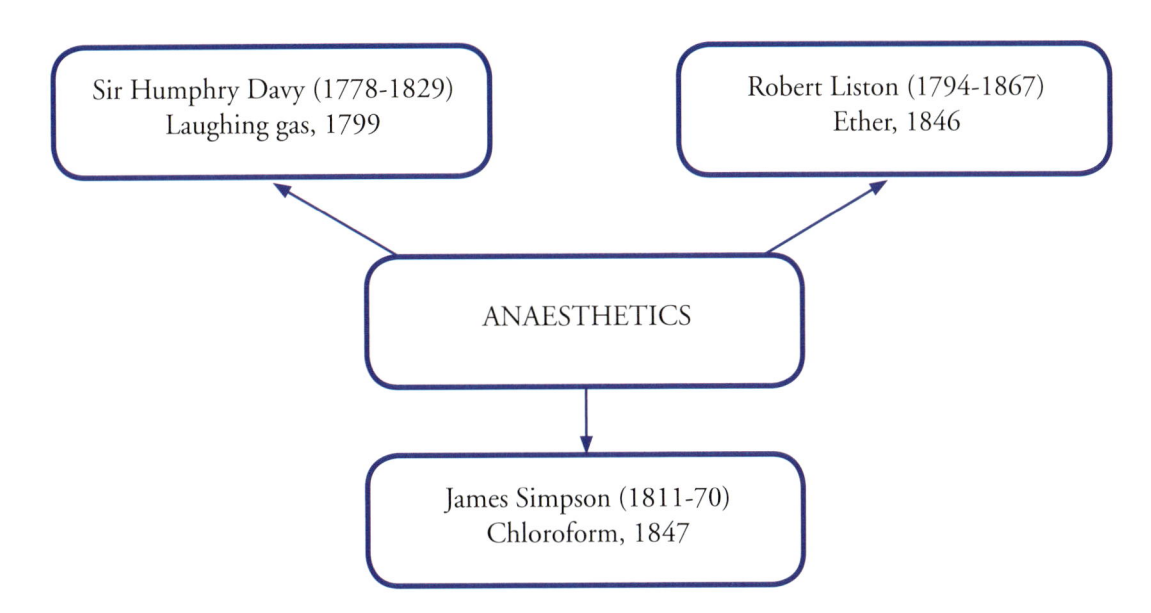

Sir Humphry Davy (1778-1829)
Laughing gas, 1799

Robert Liston (1794-1867)
Ether, 1846

ANAESTHETICS

James Simpson (1811-70)
Chloroform, 1847

SOURCE 8

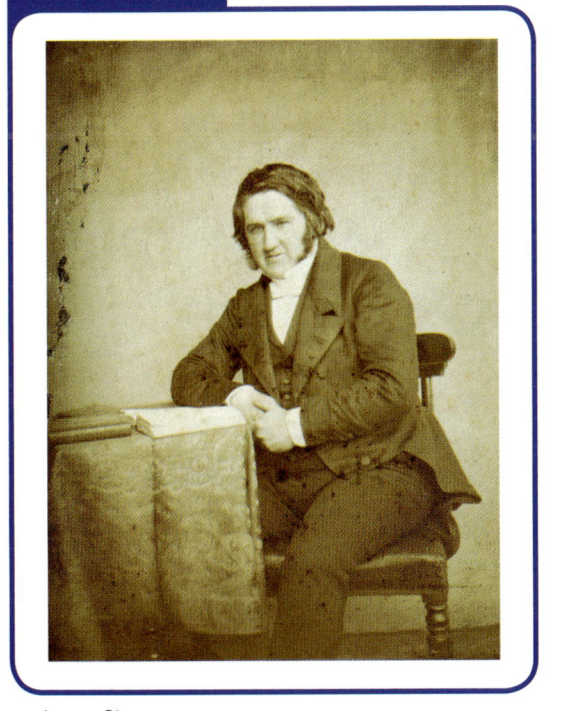

James Simpson

James Young Simpson (1811-70) was Professor of Midwifery at Edinburgh University. He was dissatisfied with using ether as an anaesthetic and so experimented with a number of other chemicals, including chloroform. He carried out a very unusual experiment, which was to have a very beneficial effect on millions of patients in the future. One evening in 1847 Simpson invited two of his friends, Dr Keith and Dr Duncan, to his home to experiment with various chemicals to see if they had any anaesthetic properties. They eventually turned to a chemical called chloroform. Simpson wrote later:

SOURCE 9

I poured some of the fluid [chloroform] into tumblers before my assistants, Dr. Keith and Dr. Duncan, and myself. Before sitting down to supper we all inhaled the fluid, and were all 'under the mahogany [table]' in a trice, to my wife's consternation and alarm.

From Sir James Simpson's Introduction of Chloroform *by His Daughter, 1894, p. 415*

Fortunately Simpson and his two colleagues eventually woke up and he realised that, in chloroform, he had discovered a very effective anaesthetic. As Professor of Midwifery, Simpson soon started using chloroform to help relieve pain during childbirth. He wrote articles about his discovery and other surgeons started to use chloroform in their operations.

SOURCE 10

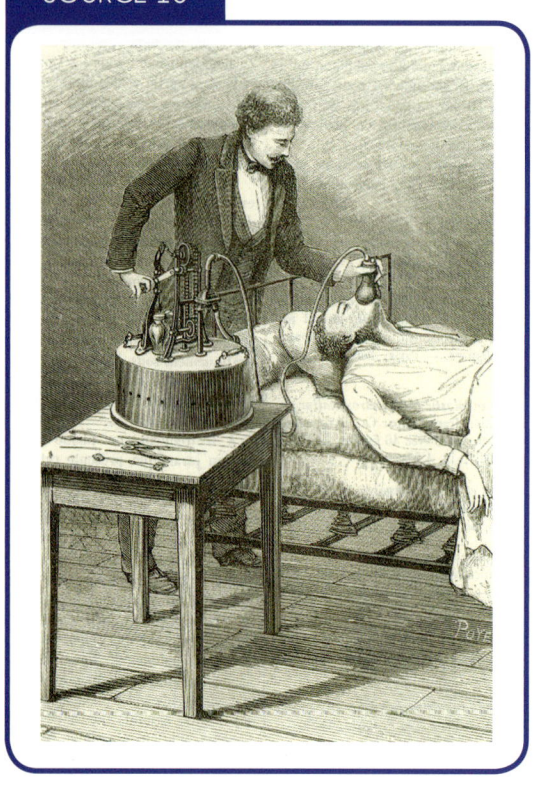

A patient inhaling chloroform

Even though chloroform had made painless operations possible, there was opposition to its use as an anaesthetic. The arguments against its use were:
- Chloroform was a new and untested gas;
- Surgeons did not know what dose to give patients;
- The first death from using chloroform occurred when Hannah Greener died during an operation in 1848 to remove her toenail. This alarmed surgeons;
- There were moral and religious arguments against the use of chloroform. One clergyman wrote that chloroform was "a decoy of Satan, apparently offering itself to bless woman, but in the end it will harden society, and rob God of the deepest cries which arise in time of trouble for help.";
- Anaesthetics did not necessarily make surgery safer as, with the patient unconscious, surgeons could carry out more complicated operations, possibly causing infection and more loss of blood.

Gradually, the use of anaesthetics was accepted, thanks to the determination of James Simpson. He had to convince colleagues and the public in general that anaesthetics were a safe option.

After a ten-year struggle, the use of anaesthetics was accepted. The final breakthrough came when Queen Victoria accepted chloroform during the birth of her eighth child, Leopold, in 1853. She was full of praise for chloroform and, from this point on, the use of anaesthetics became a standard part of surgical practice. Surgical techniques were transformed as operations could now proceed with care, rather than speed.

SOURCE 11

Previously to that time [the 16th century], surgeons had no other means of stemming the flow of blood – after amputation of the limbs for instance – than by scorching over the raw and bleeding wound with a red-hot iron, or by plunging it into boiling pitch ... [Therefore] the great and happy suggestion of Ambroise Paré ... to shut up the bleeding vessels, by constricting or tying them ... was a vast and mighty improvement. ... It saved immeasurably the sufferings of the patients, while it added immeasureably to their safety. But the practice was new, and an innovation; ... and ... like all other innovations in medical practice, it was, at first and for long, bitterly decried and denounced. ...

We look back with sorrow upon the ... opponents of Paré. In the course of years our successors in the profession will, I most sincerely believe, look back with similar feelings ... and they will equally marvel at the idea of ... humane men complacently confessing and upholding, that they prefer operating upon their patients in a waking instead of an anaesthetic state; and that the fearful agonies which they thus inflict ... should be endured ... quietly ...

All pain is ... destructive and even ultimately fatal in its action and effects.

From Remarks on the Superinduction of Anaesthesia in Natural and Morbid Parturition with Cases Illustrative of the Use and Effects of Chloroform in Obstetric Practice *by James Young Simpson, published in 1847, pp. 1, 4, 6, 10, after being read to the Medico-Chirurgical Society of Edinburgh at their meeting on 1 December that year*

SOURCE 12

With the introduction of anaesthesia the whole concept of surgery and the patient's attitude to it has changed. The prospect of undergoing a surgical operation has for most of us ceased to be a matter of stark terror, and the surgeon now looks upon an operation as a preventive measure, where previously it was performed only as a last resort.

Historian William Armstrong, writing in an article entitled 'Under the Surgeon's knife' in History Makers: The Magazine that brings History to Life, *30 January 1970*

TASKS

1. Describe in your own words Simpson's 'home experiment' with chloroform.
2. Write a list of arguments in favour of anaesthetics and a list against their use.
3. Study Source 11. Which part of the argument do you think was the strongest, in convincing doctors to use anaesthetics?

THE DEVELOPMENT OF ANTISEPTICS

The problem of pain during surgery had been addressed. The problem of infection was still a major issue. Although surgery was less painful, it was not safer. Until knowledge of the germ theory was made public in the 1860s, surgeons did not take any precautions to protect open wounds from infection.

The need for antiseptics

Infection continued to be the greatest danger to patients after an operation. Surgeons could spread infection by re-using bandages; they did not wash their hands before an operation; they did not sterilise their equipment; some surgeons operated wearing old pus-stained clothes. In fact, some patients thought that the dirtier a surgeon's coat, the more operations he must have done, so the greater the chance that they would survive if they let him operate on them.

SOURCE 13

I remember the house-surgeon ... with his ... threaded needles dangling from the front flap of his coat, ... the silken threads sweeping the well-worn cloth which had grown old in the presence of sepsis. ... One of our surgeons lectured upon anatomy in an old frock-coat ... I see it now, faded with age, stained with blood and spotted with pus

John Rudd Leeson, a colleague of Lister, remembering his time training as a surgeon, in Lister as I knew him, *1927, pp. 4-5*

Hungarian-born Dr Ignaz Semmelweis (1818-65) worked as an assistant in obstetrics in a teaching hospital in Vienna. In 1847 he observed that physicians and medical students began their day by carrying out post-mortems and then went straight to the labour wards to deliver babies. He also found that the death rate from infection was much higher amongst these women than those who had been attended by midwives, who did not carry out post-mortems. In order to cut down on the spread of infection, Dr Semmelweis insisted that all physicians and students washed their hands in a lime chloride solution before entering the wards. He was regarded as a crank and a fanatic for this, but the number of deaths at his hospital soon dropped. It was to be many years before these measures were to be adopted in Britain.

Joseph Lister (1827-1912) has been called 'the father of antiseptic surgery'. He was the son of Joseph Jackson Lister, who had developed a much-improved microscope in 1830. Lister had researched gangrene and infection and had a keen interest in applying science to medicine. He became Professor of Surgery at various universities – Glasgow (1859), Edinburgh (1869) and King's College Hospital, London (1877-93).

SOURCE 14

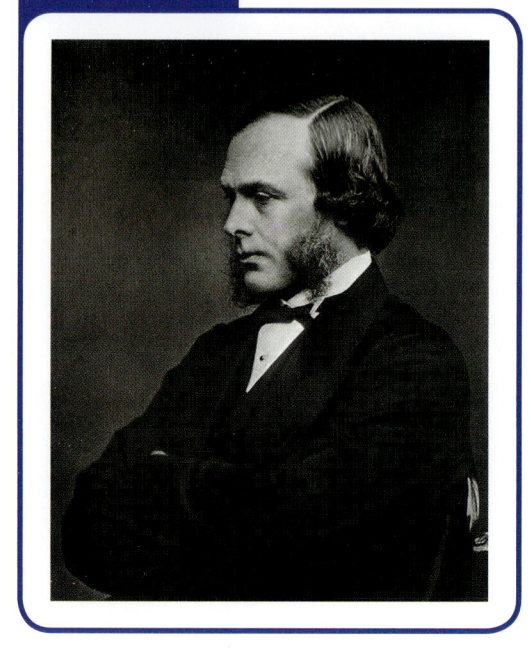

Joseph Lister

In 1865 Lister read the work of Pasteur on the germ theory, which had been published just a few years previously. This gave him an insight into how germs spread because, according to Pasteur's theory, bacteria caused disease. Unlike many other doctors at the time, Lister believed in the germ theory and tried to do something to prevent patients from dying of blood poisoning after an operation.

Lister searched for a substance that would prevent infection after surgery. He had heard that carbolic acid was being used to clean sewerage in the north of England, and decided to apply this idea to surgery. He decided to use carbolic acid to wash his hands and all of his instruments before he began any of his operations. He discovered that he could prevent wounds from becoming infected by soaking bandages in carbolic acid and wrapping them around the wounds. Lister then decided that the best way to prevent infection was to stop germs from getting to a wound in the first place. By the end of 1865 he was already insisting that bandages were used only once, that doctors and surgeons washed their hands regularly and that silk threads used for sewing up wounds were soaked in carbolic acid.

Lister had got his assistant to spray carbolic acid on the site of the patient's wound using a spray machine that he had invented himself. His methods of trying to fight infection became known as 'antiseptic surgery'.

SOURCE 15

Lister tried out his idea in a daring experiment. An 11-year-old boy called James had been run over by a cart. His leg had been broken. In the old days a surgeon might have cut off the leg, to save the boy from gangrene, a serious infection of wounds.

However, Lister decided to treat the wound with the [carbolic] spray and then to put splints on the leg. For days Lister waited to see if infection would set in. To his great delight and relief Lister found that the bone had healed up and the boy was not going to die of infection.

Historians Peter Mantin and Richard Pulley, writing in Medicine Through the Ages, *1988*

Lister published his discovery in 1867. Yet again, there was opposition to a new medical technique – in this case, the use of antiseptics in surgery. This was because:
- The carbolic spray cracked the surgeon's skin, hurt his eyes and made everything smell;
- Pasteur's ideas of the germ theory had spread very slowly. Few people understood them;
- Surgeons still believed that speed was the important thing. Lister's antiseptic methods slowed things down;

SOURCE 16

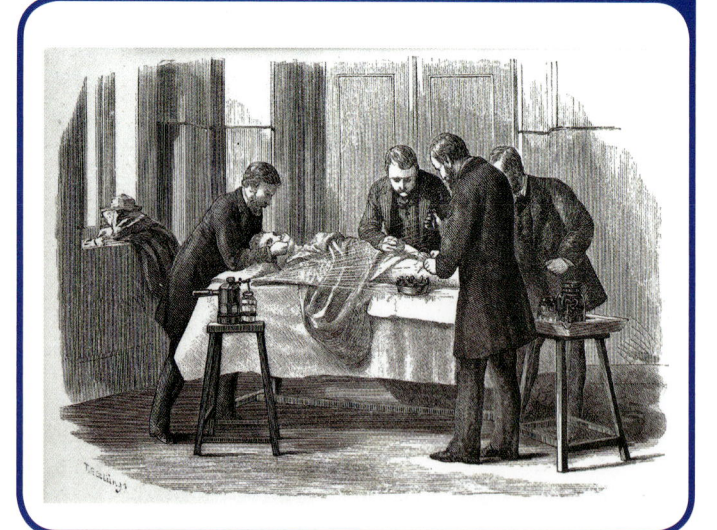

An operation using carbolic spray

- For centuries surgeons had become accustomed to the fact that lots of their patients would die anyway. When Lister said that he had kept his patients alive, other surgeons refused to believe him;

SOURCE 17

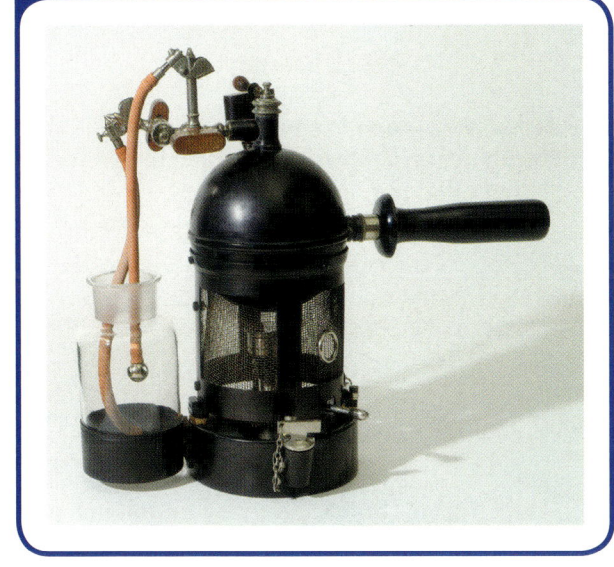

A carbolic steam spray 1872-1887

- When some surgeons copied Lister's methods, they got poorer results because they were less systematic and less careful;
- Lister appeared to be cold, arrogant and aloof. He sometimes criticised other surgeons, so they turned against him;
- Lister kept changing his techniques. His critics accused him of changing his methods because they did not work.

Despite the opposition, Lister's methods marked a turning point in surgery. In 1877 he moved from Glasgow to London, as Professor of Surgery at King's College Hospital. In 1878 Robert Koch discovered the bacterium that caused septicaemia (blood poisoning) and this gave Lister's ideas a great boost. By the late 1890s his antiseptic methods – which killed germs on the wound – had led to **aseptic surgery**. This meant removing all possible germs from the operating theatre. To ensure complete cleanliness, various measures were introduced:

- Operating theatres were thoroughly cleaned;
- From 1887 all surgical instruments were steam-sterilised;
- In 1894 sterilised rubber gloves (first used by the US surgeon, William Halstead) were used in Britain for the first time.

In 1892, Lister and Pasteur were given an award at the Sorbonne University in Paris in recognition of their contribution to the fight against disease. Towards the end of his life Lister was made a Lord and his contribution to surgical methods is so important that surgery is now divided into two periods of time – *before* Lister and *after* Lister. When he died in 1912 the Royal College of Surgeons paid this tribute to Joseph Lister:

> "His work will last for all time. Humanity will bless him evermore and his fame will be immortal."

With two of the basic problems of surgery – pain and infection – now solved, surgeons could attempt more ambitious operations. The increased ease and safety of surgery stimulated the beginnings of surgical specialisation. The first successful operation to remove an infected appendix took place in the 1880s. The first heart operation was carried out in 1896 when surgeons repaired a heart damaged by a stab wound.

However, a continuing problem during surgery was how to stop bleeding. Lister also made a contribution here. He improved on traditional ligatures by using sterilised catgut that did not pose such a great risk of infection as silk thread. Other surgeons experimented with blood transfusion, but with little success. It wasn't until 1901 that scientists discovered that there were different blood groups and that transfusion only worked if the donor's blood group matched that of the receiver.

TASKS

1. Do some research. What was the contribution of Dr Ignaz Semmelweis to surgery?
2. How did Pasteur's germ theory help develop Lister's ideas?
3. Draw a spider-type diagram to show the opposition to Lister's ideas on antiseptics.
4. How successful was Joseph Lister?

Orthopaedics and the 'Anglesey Bonesetter'

SOURCE 18

One dark, stormy night about 1743, a ship is said to have become wrecked off the treacherous north Anglesey coast.

The only survivors of that wreck ... were two [young] boys ...

They were said to speak an unknown language.

'Where had they come from?'

The geographical origins of the boys has long been a mystery, with notions of a Spanish nationality ...

One of the boys ... died soon after his rescue. The other, now named Evan Thomas by his adoptive family in Llanfairynghornwy, flourished and demonstrated a remarkable ability at healing the broken bones of animals. Evan later applied his great skill to human bones, and became much sought-after ... Evan's later descendants became fully-qualified doctors and spawned [started] a new branch of medicine we now call orthopaedics.

The most famous of Evan's descendants was Hugh Owen Thomas (1834-91). Hugh was born at Bodedern in Anglesey, and became known as Meddyg Esgyrn (the Bone Doctor). Hugh first trained with his uncle, Dr Owen Roberts, at St Asaph in North Wales before studying medicine at Edinburgh and at University College, London. He qualified as a surgeon in 1857 and set up a practice in Liverpool.

Hugh Owen Thomas' greatest contribution was to orthopaedics. He developed the 'Thomas Splint', which was used to stabilise a fractured thigh bone and to prevent infection. The Thomas splint, sometimes referred to simply as 'the Thomas' was often used in the First World War and its basic design is still used today.

From an Internet website (www.angleseybonesetters.co.uk)

SOURCE 19

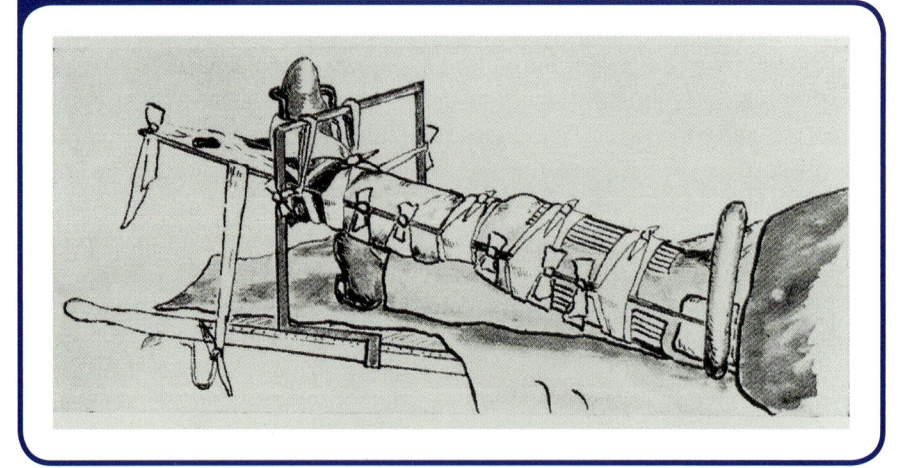

The Thomas splint

TASK

Do some research and describe the achievement of the Thomas family of Anglesey.

Examination practice

This section provides guidance on how to answer Question 1(d), 2(d) and 3(d) from Unit 3. The question is worth 8 marks.

Question 1(d), 2(d), 3(d) – the selection of own knowledge and the analysis of key concepts

How important was the work of James Simpson in improving surgery in the nineteenth century?

[8 marks]

Tips on how to answer

- This type of question requires you to **evaluate the importance** (sometimes the question will refer to **success**) of a particular event, movement or individual.
- You must aim to **analyse and evaluate** the reasons for this importance/success.
- Descriptive answers will not score you more than half marks – **you must analyse**.
- You need to support your observations with **specific factual detail.**
- Remember that this question requires you to **provide a judgement**, giving specific reasons why you think this event, movement or individual was important or successful.

Response by candidate one

James Simpson was Professor of Midwifery. He and his colleagues experimented with different chemicals; when they inhaled chloroform, they passed out! Simpson realised that he had discovered a very effective anaesthetic. He soon started using chloroform to relieve women's labour pains during childbirth. Other surgeons started to use chloroform during their operations.

Examiner's comment

Although the answer is accurate, it lacks factual detail. It is a mostly descriptive answer, which hints at the importance of Simpson's work, but the judgement is not fully sustained. The answer is worth low Level Two (4 marks).

Response by candidate two

James Simpson was Professor of Midwifery at Edinburgh University. Operations at the time were painful processes and he wanted to find a way of making surgery less painful. One evening in 1847, he invited two of his colleagues to his home to experiment with some chemicals that could reduce the feeling of pain. When they inhaled chloroform, they passed out. Simpson realised that this could be a very effective anaesthetic to relieve pain during operations.

Simpson soon used chloroform as an anaesthetic, to relieve women's labour pains during childbirth. He wrote articles about his discovery and other surgeons started to use chloroform during their operations. With the use of chloroform as an anaesthetic, operations could now be painless, longer and more complex.

There was initial opposition to Simpson's use of chloroform, so his work was not immediately important. Chloroform was a new and untested gas; surgeons did not know what dose to give patients; a patient died in 1848, undergoing an operation using chloroform; and there were moral and religious oppositions to the use of chloroform at that time. The struggle to recognise the importance of using chloroform as an anaesthetic in surgery went on for ten years until, in 1853, Queen Victoria accepted the use of chloroform during the delivery of her eighth child. Anaesthetics then became a standard part of surgical practice and surgery became generally safer due to the work of James Simpson in the nineteenth century.

Examiner's comment

This is a detailed, accurate and well-structured answer. The candidate addresses the key issue throughout. A reasoned judgement is made and the answer addresses the thrust of the question. The answer meets the requirements of Level Three and is worthy of receiving maximum (8) marks.

Now you have a go

How important was the work of Joseph Lister in improving surgery in the nineteenth century?

[8 marks]

CHAPTER 6

WHAT HAVE BEEN THE MAIN TURNING POINTS IN THE PREVENTION AND TREATMENT OF DISEASE FROM THE TWENTIETH CENTURY TO TODAY?

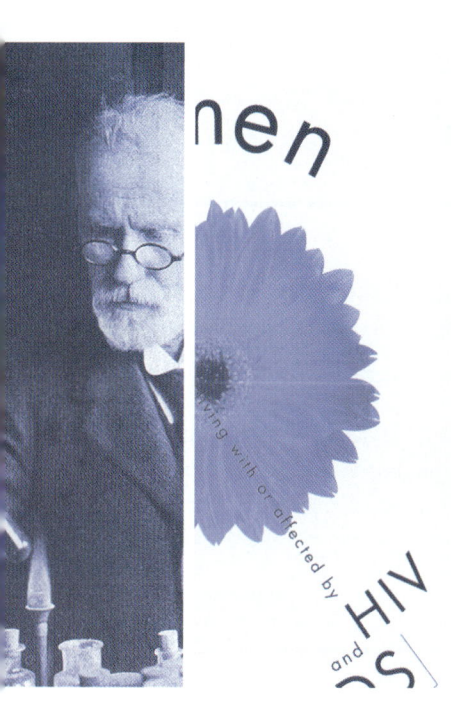

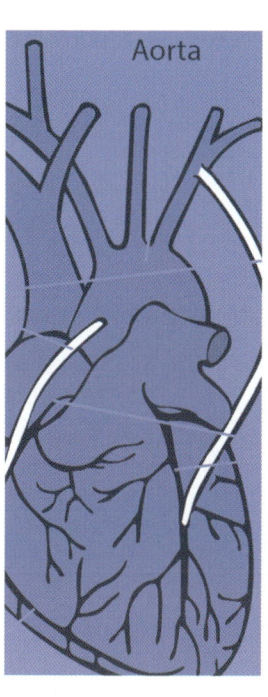

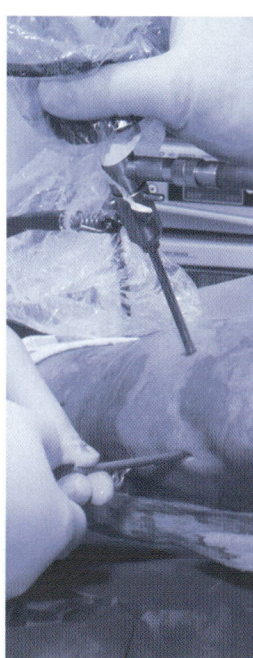

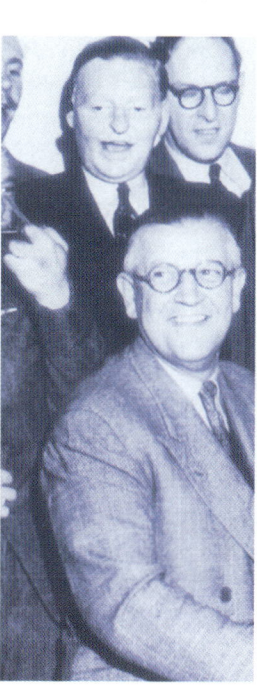

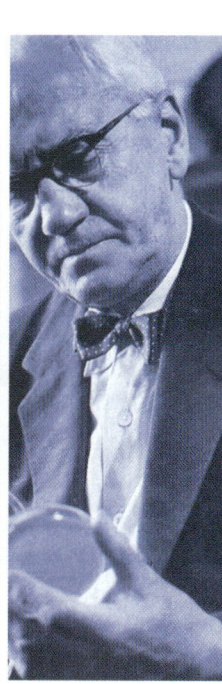

The work of Pasteur and Koch during the nineteenth century had focused on the prevention of disease. A cure for diseases was still sought at the beginning of the twentieth century and scientists tried to find chemicals that could do this work.

We have seen in Chapter 3 that scientists had started to seek out the first cures for diseases in the mid nineteenth century. Emil Behring (1854-1917) had discovered that the body produces anti-toxins that fight harmful bacteria. He had used natural means to make this discovery and to find a cure for diphtheria.

In 1891, Paul Ehrlich (1854-1915) joined Robert Koch's research team at the Infectious Diseases Institute. Koch had found that dyes could stain certain bacteria and make them easier to see, but he had not made much progress in his research. Ehrlich was fascinated by dyes and, as he carried on Koch's work, his research led him to discover that the blood contains antibodies that kill particular germs. He called these 'magic bullets' because they sought out the germs they wanted to kill without harming the rest of the human body.

THE DEVELOPMENT OF ANTIBIOTICS

The search was now on to create synthetic (man-made) chemicals for treating disease. The pharmaceutical industry was well established at this time and the discovery of a chemical wonder drug, or magic bullet could lead to massive profits. Ehrlich was one of the outstanding figures of twentieth century medical science and was a pioneer of the science of chemotherapy – the use of chemicals to destroy disease-causing organisms.

Ehrlich and his team worked for years in search of this magic bullet, but with little success. The team was trying to find a cure for a disease called syphilis.

SOURCE 1

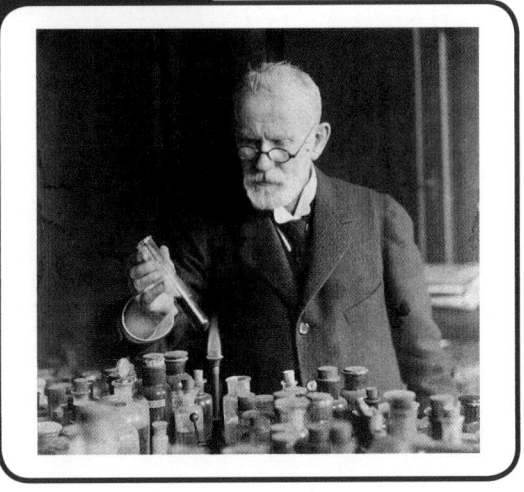

Paul Ehrlich working in his laboratory

Their task seemed impossible until Ehrlich decided to experiment with a variety of chemical compounds based on arsenic. In 1909, after experimenting with hundreds of different compounds, Dr Sahachirō Hata, a new member of Ehrlich's research team, went back to compound 606. He found that it killed the micro-organism that caused syphilis. Dr Hata described the amazing discovery:

SOURCE 2

Having made his first experiments Dr. Hata came to show Ehrlich his records and said, with his usual polite bows:

'Only first trials – only preliminary general view. ...

[Dr. Hata] 'Believe 606 *very* efficacious ...'

Ehrlich looked at the records and said, much astonished:

'No, surely not? ... It was all minutely tested by Dr. R., and *he* found nothing – nothing! ...

[Ehrlich] 'More than a year ago we laid aside 606 as being ineffective, worthless. You are sure you are not mistaken, Dr. Hata?'

Hata pointed to the records of the experiments and said, shrugging his shoulders:

'I found *that*, Herr Geheimrat.'

'Then it must be repeated, dear Hata, repeated,' said Ehrlich. ...

One morning he [Ehrlich] came quickly into his laboratory, followed by Dr. Hata, who had been waiting for him, with his record books. ...

'Well, my dear Hata, what have you found out now?' asked Ehrlich, coming near.

With repeated nods of his head, Dr. Hata replied:

'Always – 606 best!'

'Incredible!' ... said Ehrlich. 'What an incapable good-for-nothing!' he exclaimed, his big eyes looking at Dr. Hata over the tops of his spectacles. Hata looked scared and stretched out his arms as if in defence. Ehrlich put his hand on Hata's shoulder, soothingly, and shook his head. 'Oh, not *you*,' he said, '*not you!* No, the other fellow before you,' he went on disgustedly. ' ... der ungeschickte Taperkerl!' (the stupid good-for-nothing!).

Then Dr. Hata beamed with delight and grinning broadly, he repeated, 'Ungeschickte Taperkerl!'

Herr Geheimrat: an honorary title given to exceptional scientists

From Martha Marquardt's biography, Paul Ehrlich, *1951*

The new drug was named Salvarsan, or sometimes just 606, and was released in 1910. It was soon sold all over the world. The discovery was a turning point, since this was the first synthetic chemical compound that had been used successfully to destroy micro-organisms. The first man-made magic bullet had been found. The discovery of Salvarsan inspired other researchers to continue with their search for other magic bullets that could cure different diseases.

SOURCE 3

The success of Salvarsan before and during the First World War had demonstrated that microbes could be destroyed by synthetic drugs that did not damage the [host] ..., but the search for similar ... drugs was not particularly successful.

Historian E. M. Tansey, writing in Western Medicine: An Illustrated History, *1997*

The First World War had interrupted the research into synthetic drugs but, in the 1920s, research started again, albeit very slowly. In 1932 Gerhardt Domagk (1895-1964) was working in the Bayer Pharmaceutical Laboratories in Germany when he discovered that a dye called Prontosil Red destroyed the bacteria that caused blood poisoning in mice, without any ill effects on the mice.

Prontosil needed to be tested on a human and the opportunity arose sooner than Domagk expected, when his daughter accidentally pricked her finger on an infected needle in his laboratory and developed severe blood poisoning. When she was near to death, Domagk decided that the only way to save her was to inject her with the previously untried Prontosil. This was a great risk but the girl recovered and survived. A second magic bullet had been found.

Gerhardt Domagk won the Nobel Prize for Medicine in 1939 'for the discovery of the antibacterial effects of Prontosil'.

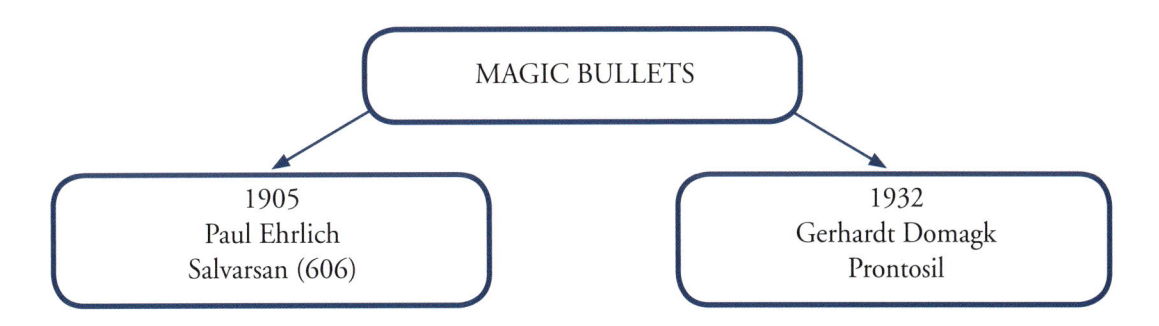

```
              MAGIC BULLETS
              /            \
       1905                   1932
       Paul Ehrlich           Gerhardt Domagk
       Salvarsan (606)        Prontosil
```

The next step was to find out what the active ingredient was in Prontosil. Clinical trials took place in the UK at Queen Charlotte's Maternity Hospital and in Paris. In 1934 it was announced that the active ingredient was a sulphonamide, derived from coal tar. The discovery of sulphonamides had been accomplished very quickly with the aid of a powerful electron microscope that had been invented in 1931.

Soon companies all around the world manufactured sulphonamides and soon there was a race on to discover cures based on this group of chemicals. This was a period of great excitement and activity. Sulphonamides were immediately of vital importance in counteracting **puerperal fever** (also known as childbed fever – a deadly bacterial infection caught by many women during childbirth), scarlet fever, meningitis, pneumonia and gonorrhoea.

These new drugs were introduced into clinical practice in the late 1930s and they soon helped to improve health. **Maternal mortality** was reduced because infections following the birth of a child could now be controlled. Although largely replaced today by antibiotics, sulphonamides still play a role in antibacterial chemotherapy, and their discovery was important in opening up new possibilities in medical cures. However, it was the discovery of the first real antibiotic that was to be a major turning point in the treatment of disease.

TASKS

1. Describe the work of Paul Ehrlich.
2. How important was Salvarsan?
3. How successful was the work of Gerhardt Domagk?

Alexander Fleming and penicillin

There were still many germs that could not be killed, even with sulphonamides. During the First World War thousands of soldiers had died when minor wounds became septic. There was no reliable way of killing the germs that often infected wounds received on the battlefield.

The answer to the problem was found in the penicillin mould. This was the first of the so-called 'wonder drugs', because it killed many different bacteria. John Sanderson first discovered penicillin in the early nineteenth century. In the 1880s Joseph Lister rediscovered Sanderson's work and successfully used penicillin to treat a young nurse with an infected wound. However, he did not leave any notes or details of his methods. Other scientists also investigated penicillin, but were unable to produce sufficient quantities to be of much use.

Alexander Fleming (1881-1955) was a Scottish bacteriologist. He worked at St Mary's Hospital, Paddington, in London. He was the first person to use anti-typhoid vaccines on human beings and he also pioneered the **intravenous** use of Salvarsan against syphilis.

SOURCE 4

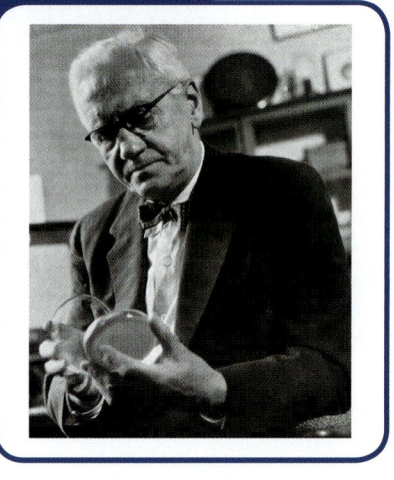

Sir Alexander Fleming in his laboratory

During the First World War, Fleming served as a medical officer in France. There he saw thousands of soldiers die of infected wounds. This made him determined to find a way to treat infection when he left the army in 1918. For the next ten years Fleming carried out countless experiments in his laboratory at St Mary's Hospital. It was here, in 1928, that he re-discovered the properties of penicillin.

SOURCE 5

In this laboratory Fleming grew bacteria on small plates and tested them to see if they killed germs. Although he tried thousands of plates, none of them seemed to work. Then, one day in 1928, just before his summer holidays, he began some more experiments. Because it was so hot he left the window open. He went away. When he returned to the laboratory he quickly checked the plates to see what had happened to them. He was not very hopeful. Nothing special seemed to have happened to them and he decided to wash them up and start again. Suddenly, to his surprise he noticed a huge blob on one of the plates. The blob seemed to have killed the germs around it. This was just what he had been looking for!

He grew some more of the mould, called Penicillium Notatum, and realised that it killed many different germs. However, he found it difficult to grow large amounts of the mould

Historians Peter Mantin and Richard Pulley, writing in Medicine Through the Ages, *1997*

In Fleming's experiment, the penicillin had killed the staphylococcus bacteria. When he grew more of the Penicillium notatum mould, he found that it killed many different bacteria. Through continued experimentation, he found that penicillin could be applied to or injected into areas infected with penicillin-sensitive micro-organisms. Fleming had in fact discovered a substance with unrivalled anti-biotic powers. However, he did not have the facilities or the support to develop and test his idea that penicillin could fight infection. As yet, there was no means of producing this drug on a large scale. All that Fleming could do at this point was to publish a report in 1929 on his outstanding discovery.

Fleming had to wait for more than a decade before two brilliant experimental scientists at Oxford University, Howard Florey and Ernst Chain, perfected a method of mass producing penicillin. Fleming carried on his work at St Mary's Hospital where he became Professor of Bacteriology in 1938. Along with Florey and Chain, he was awarded the Nobel Prize for Medicine in 1945.

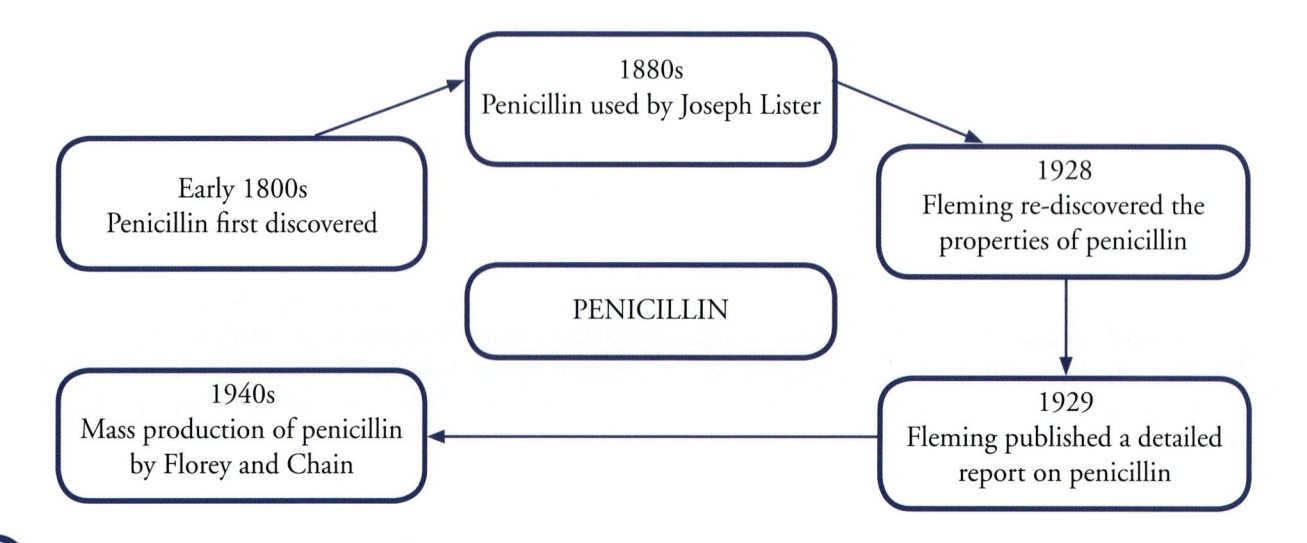

PENICILLIN

- Early 1800s: Penicillin first discovered
- 1880s: Penicillin used by Joseph Lister
- 1928: Fleming re-discovered the properties of penicillin
- 1929: Fleming published a detailed report on penicillin
- 1940s: Mass production of penicillin by Florey and Chain

Florey and Chain and the mass production of penicillin

From a medical point of view, the Second World War (1939-1945) created as many problems as the First World War. With many thousands of soldiers being injured, the medical system came under severe pressure. The lack of availability of natural products put enormous pressure on the pharmaceutical industry. The mass production of Fleming's antibacterial wonder drug – penicillin – became an urgent necessity.

SOURCE 6

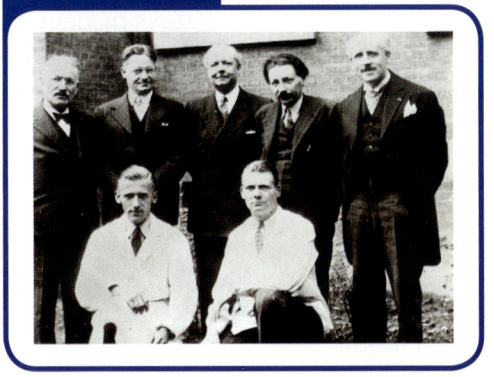

Howard Florey (back row, 2nd from left) and Ernst Chain (back row, 2nd from right) with a group of visiting VIPs who came to see the Oxford team's work

Australian-born Howard Florey (1898-1968) and German-born Ernst Chain (1906-79) worked together at the biochemistry department at Oxford University and had both become interested in Fleming's 1929 report on penicillin. In 1939, at the very start of the Second World War, they assembled a skilled research team and applied to the British government for money to fund the team's research into the drug.

SOURCE 7

I enclose some proposals which ... have a very practical bearing at the moment.
    There are ... accounts ... of substances with chemical properties ...which act powerfully on pathogenic bacteria, ... These substances have been obtained from ... strains of penicillium, ...
    Filtrates of certain strains of penicillium contain a ... substance, called penicillin by its discoverer Fleming, which is especially effective against [certain bacteria] ... the properties of penicillin ... hold out promise of its finding a practical application in the treatment of ... infections.
    In view of the possible great practical importance of the above ... it is proposed to prepare these substances in a purified form suitable for intravenous injection and to study their antiseptic action *in vivo*.

Part of Florey's proposal to the Medical Research Council, 6 September 1939

Florey and Chain were successful in their application for money. They now had to go through three stages in the development of their work:
- Grow the penicillin in sufficient quantities to test;
- Test the penicillin on animals – they did this on mice;
- Carry out trials on humans.

By early 1941, the research team had produced enough penicillin for a human trial.

SOURCE 8

Well, the Radcliffe Infirmary like all hospitals had a septic ward. And I went down there to find somebody who had a serious infection with a germ, which could not be cured by other drugs but penicillin might cure. And there was a policeman there [Albert Alexander].
... A delightful man who'd been in having ... septicaemia, with boils breaking out all over him. He'd lost one eye from being poisoned. He had boils all over him, and he was in a desperate state. And we started penicillin. And it was absolutely miraculous! The next day, he said, for the first time he was feeling better. His temperature came down. And so it went on for four, five days. And then the supply of the penicillin was so scarce that I used to collect his urine in the evening each day, and bicycle with it over to the Dunn Laboratory, where Chain and Florey would be waiting to hear the latest clinical news. And I would give them this urine, and they would extract the penicillin so that the patient could have on the third day the same penicillin he'd had on the first day. But in spite of this ... on the third or fourth day, the penicillin ran out, and it hadn't completely cured his infection. The poor man, the poor man then deteriorated and died about a week later

Professor Charles Fletcher, a member of Florey's research team, in an interview with Max Blythe at Oxford, June 1984

Although the test-patient died, the trial confirmed that penicillin was a powerful drug and that Florey and Chain and their research team had successfully isolated and purified for clinical use the anti-bacterial substance, penicillin. Florey was convinced that if enough penicillin had been available the test-patient would have survived.

The production of penicillin continued to be frustratingly slow but, as more was produced, two more patients were treated successfully. Florey even used penicillin to treat a friend who had meningitis. The wonder drug was beginning to prove itself.

The increasing number of British casualties in the Second World War meant that the mass production of penicillin was now becoming more and more important, so that this powerful new drug could be put to use. Florey knew that a lot of research and investment were necessary to produce the amount of penicillin needed for effective use at this time.

Despite considerable efforts in Britain through the work of the major pharmaceutical companies, co-operating as the Therapeutic Research Corporation, the quantities of penicillin being produced still weren't enough. The threat of German bomings was also an obstacle to mass production in Britain, so in June 1941 Florey travelled to the USA to try to get drug companies there interested in its dvelopment. At first, he was treated with suspicion. However, when the USA entered the Second World War in December 1941, after the Japanese attack on the American naval base at Pearl Harbour, the situation changed completely.

- In 1942 the American government gave $80 million to four drug companies to find a way to mass produce penicillin;
- In 1943 production began and penicillin was first used by the British Army in North Africa;
- By the time of the D Day invasion in June 1944 there was enough penicillin to treat all of the casualties;
- By 1945 the American army was using two million doses of penicillin a month. Numerous lives were saved and the time that the infected wounded spent in hospital was cut dramatically.

Soon after the Second World War ended in 1945, penicillin became available for civilian use. It was commonly known as an antibiotic. The eventual success of penicillin, together with the pre-war use of sulphonamides, meant the beginning of the 'antibiotic era'. War, government action and scientific research and discoveries all contributed to the production of this 'wonder drug' of the twentieth century.

SOURCE 9

'We had an enormous number of infected wounded,' says Pulvertaft, 'terrible burn cases among the crews of the naval armoured cars, and fractures infected with streptococci. ... the sulphonamides ... had absolutely no effect on these cases. The last thing I tried was penicillin. I had very little of it ... The first man I tried it on was a young New Zealand officer ... He had been in bed for six months with compound fractures in both legs. His sheets were saturated with pus and the heat in Cairo made the smell intolerable. He was little more than skin and bone and was running a high temperature. Normally, he would have died in a very short while ... We introduced small rubber tubes into the sinuses of the left leg and injected with a very weak solution of penicillin ... because we had so little. I gave three injections a day and studied the effects under the microscope. ... the thing seemed like a miracle. In ten days the left leg was cured, and in a month's time the young fellow was back on his feet. I had enough penicillin left for ten cases. Nine of them were complete cures.'

A description by Lieutenant-Colonel Pulvertaft, a bacteriologist working in Egypt, of the first use of penicillin by the British Army
From The Life of Sir Alexander Fleming: Discoverer of Penicillin *by André Maurois, 1959*

TASKS

1. Use Sources 4 and 5 to show how scientific methods helped to develop penicillin.
2. Explain why the work of Florey and Chain was important.
3. Why do you think that penicillin has been called a 'wonder drug'?
4. Describe the inter-connected causes that led to the production of penicillin.

DEVELOPMENTS IN TRANSPLANT SURGERY

Of all recent developments in the field of medicine, the transplanting of human organs is perhaps the most remarkable. The development of transplant surgery was a slow process and followed on from techniques used in reconstructive surgery, pioneered in the treatment of various battle injuries in the major conflicts of the twentieth century.

Airmen in the Battle of Britain in 1940 suffered from a new condition, known as '**Airman's Burn**'. During the Second World War, 4,500 airmen were rescued and 80% of them had burns of the hands and face. Many were treated at the Maxillo-Facial Unit of the Queen Victoria Hospital at East Grinstead in Sussex. Here they were under the care of New Zealand-born Sir Archibald McIndoe (1900-60), who was consultant plastic surgeon to the RAF.

The Battle of Britain highlighted the need for skilled plastic surgeons, as burns from blazing aviation fuel went deep, with the problem of disfigurement and loss of function if the burnt area was not treated early. Sir Archibald was highly influential in the field of reconstructive surgery, which involves rebuilding patients using tissue from their own body, and used his skills of cutting, grafting and reconstruction to treat the burn injuries of 649 airmen. In 1941 the RAF patients on whom McIndoe had operated formed The Guinea Pig Club. They were so-called because they had acted as 'guinea pigs' in trials for many of his pioneering techniques.

SOURCE 10

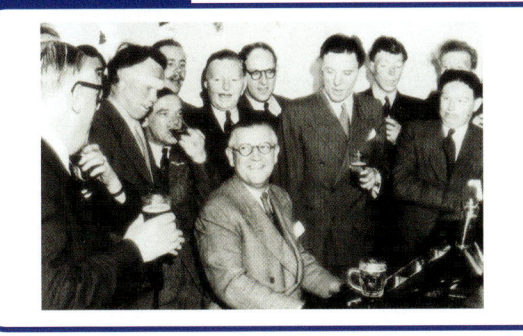

Sir Archibald McIndoe (centre) and members of the RAF 'Guinea Pig Club'

Sir Archibald never carried out transplant surgery between patients, although he had discussed the idea with another prominent surgeon of the time, his cousin Sir Harold Gillies. However, he did foresee developments in organ and reconstructive transplantation: "The next great era in surgery will be when we learn how to transplant tissue from one person to another. I foresee the day when whole limbs, kidneys, lungs and even hearts will be surgically replaced." Sir Archibald McIndoe died unexpectedly in 1960, at the age of 60 and The Blond McIndoe Research Foundation was set up in his name, which carried out research into transplantation work in its early days, but now focuses on using a patient's own cells to heal their wounds.

McIndoe's predictions came true when the first kidney transplant was carried out in the USA in the early 1950s and in the UK in 1960. Removing a kidney was a fairly easy process and, should the operation fail, the patient could be kept alive through kidney dialysis, as dialysis machines had been developed in the 1940s.

Kidney transplants immediately raised two major issues:
- Rejection of the transplanted organ;
- The availability of replacement organs.

These problems would restrict developments in the field of heart transplantation.

Heart surgery at first concentrated on repairing valves that were faulty at birth or had been damaged by subsequent illnesses. The earliest example of an operation on a damaged heart valve was in 1925. However, there was little progress in further, more complex heart surgery until more effective drugs were developed to relax patients' muscles during respiration and until the heart-lung machine was developed in 1953. This machine was able to take over the circulation and oxygenation of the blood (particularly to the brain), allowing the heart to be stopped and giving the surgeon time to work on the inactive heart.

In the 1960s heart bypass surgery was pioneered to treat coronary artery disease, which occurs when the artery walls thicken preventing blood flow to the heart muscle. The procedure involves taking lengths of the patient's own blood vessels (usually from the leg) and sewing them into the heart muscle to allow blood to flow around the blockage.

SOURCE 11

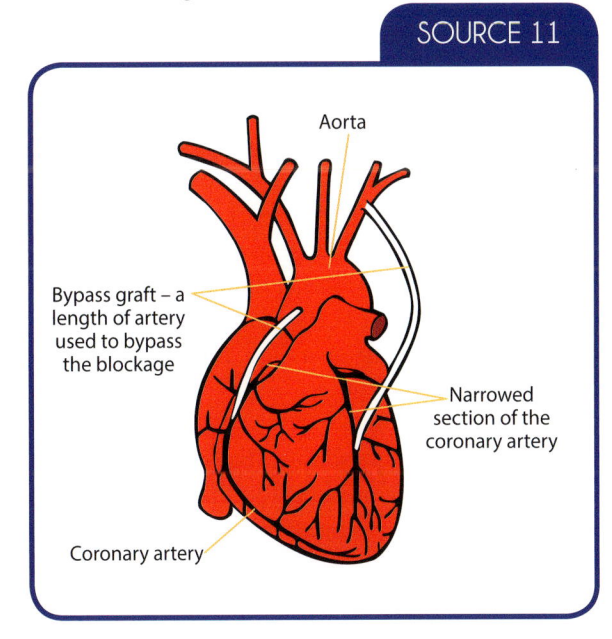

Diagram showing heart bypass

The increasing complexity of heart surgery culminated in the transplantation of a whole heart by Dr Christiaan Barnard in South Africa in 1967.

Christiaan Barnard and heart transplants

SOURCE 12

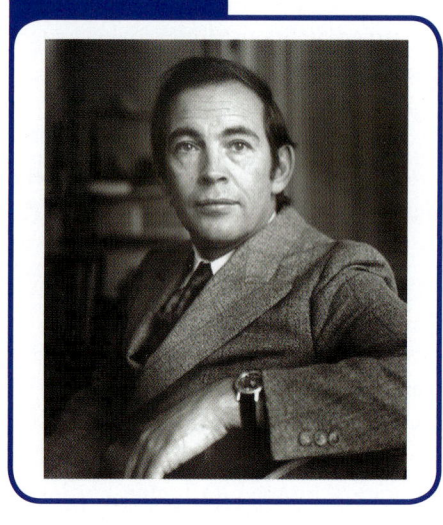

Dr Christiaan Barnard, who carried out the first heart transplant

Christiaan Barnard (1922-2001) was born in Cape Province, South Africa. One of his four brothers died of a heart problem at the age of five. This may have inspired Barnard to follow a career in medicine, which he studied at the University of Cape Town Medical School, graduating in 1945.

From 1956 to 1958 Barnard studied and worked at the University of Minnesota in the USA. There he became acquainted with pioneering research work on heart transplantation. On returning to South Africa in 1958, Barnard worked at the Groote Schuur Hospital in Cape Town. He established the hospital's first heart unit, developing a reputation as a brilliant surgeon and as an expert in the treatment of heart diseases.

In October 1967 Barnard performed the first kidney transplant in South Africa. He had experimented for several years with animal heart transplants and more than 50 dogs had received transplanted hearts. With several surgical teams at the ready Barnard now prepared for a human heart transplant; he had a patient willing to undergo the operation, but needed a suitable donor.

Christiaan Barnard performed the first human heart transplant on 3 December 1967. The operation lasted for nine hours and a team of thirty people was used. The patient was Louis Washansky, a 54-year old grocer who was suffering from diabetes and incurable heart disease. The donor heart came from a young woman, Denise Darvall, who had been declared brain damaged following an accident on 2 December, while crossing a street in Cape Town. Washansky survived the operation but lived for only 18 days, eventually dying of pneumonia.

Although Louis Washansky – the first patient to receive the heart of another human being – survived for only a short time, a turning point had been reached in transplant surgery. Barnard performed a second heart transplant operation on 2 January 1968. The patient was Philip Blaiberg; he survived for 594 days. Dorothy Fisher was given a new heart in 1969 and became the first black person to receive a heart transplant; she lived for 12 years and six months after the operation. Dirk Van Zyl received a new heart in 1971 and lived for a further 23 years. (In Britain, the longest-lived heart transplant patient was Derrick Morris, who received a new heart in February 1980 and died in August 2005.)

Barnard performed ten heart transplants between 1967 and 1973. Many surgeons gave up heart transplants because of poor results, as the new organs were often rejected. Barnard persisted with his pioneering work until the development of the **immunosuppressive agent**, cyclosporine, meant that transplanted organs were less likely to be rejected. The use of this agent revived interest in heart transplant surgery, so that the procedure has now become fairly common.

Christiaan Barnard became world famous for his pioneering work. He had established heart transplant surgery as a successful procedure and this led to many more types of transplant surgery becoming possible – lungs, liver, pancreas, corneas and even faces.

Modern transplant surgery

Many transplant procedures were unsuccessful because of the problem of rejection. The use of immunosuppressive drugs helped solve this particular problem, but the lack of sufficient human organs for transplantation is still an issue. In the early 1950s French surgeons had used kidneys from executed criminals. However, the usual source of organs is patients who have been declared 'brain dead'.

This has led to public debates in many countries about the ethical issues of organ donation. However, by the mid-1980s, many countries had established nationwide, or even continent-wide, transplant programmes. Records are now kept of potential recipients for heart and lungs, for liver and pancreas, and for kidneys. In Wales today, the Welsh Government has raised the issue of whether there should be an opt-out system for organ donation, rather than the present opt-in system. This is a very contentious issue and reflects the fact that developments in transplant surgery have out-paced the availability of donor organs.

> **TASKS**
>
> 1. Why do you think that Sir Archibald McIndoe could be called a 'visionary'?
> 2. Study Source 11. Briefly describe heart bypass surgery in your own words.
> 3. Why was the heart operation performed by Dr Christiaan Barnard in 1967 a turning point in transplant surgery?

MODERN DRUGS AND TREATMENT

In the early twenty first century the terrifying diseases of earlier centuries are no longer the main causes of death. A combination of antibiotics, immunisations and public health measures has conquered them. Today illnesses such as cancer and heart disease are responsible for the majority of deaths.

SOURCE 13

non-infectious diseases, like cancers and cardiovascular [heart] diseases, have soared into prominence on the lists of causes of death. ... [they] are posing enormous problems for the health services of many countries ... These are the epidemics of the modern Western world.

Historian Mary Dobson, writing in Western Medicine: An Illustrated History, *1997*

Cancer

Cancer is the uncontrolled growth of cells in parts of the human body. If these cancer cells split off and move into vital organs such as the kidneys or liver, secondary cancers can grow there. Very often it is these secondary cancers that cause death. Cancerous growths start because a change occurs in the DNA of a cell. Despite extensive research over recent decades, scientists still do not know exactly what causes this change. However, it is known that skin cancer can be triggered by sunburn, bowel cancer by unhealthy diet and lung cancer by smoking.

Although quite rare at one time, lung cancer is now the most common cancer amongst British men and its frequency is increasing in women too. The major cause of lung cancer, as shown as far back as 1950, is cigarette smoking. Yet, despite the evidence, publicity and health warnings, people continue to smoke – and to die of lung cancer.

SOURCE 14

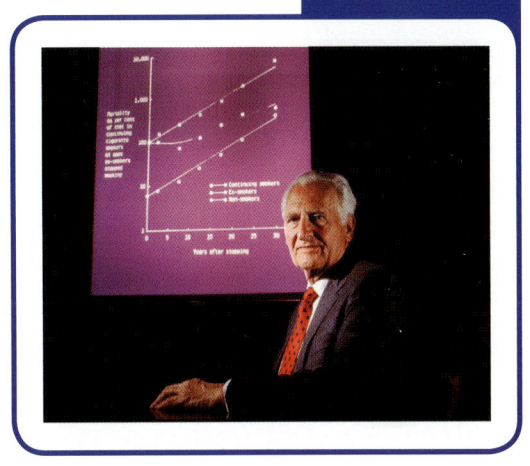

Sir Richard Shaboe Doll (1912-2005), British physiologist, with a graph from his study on the mortality associated with cigarette smoking. Doll was a pioneer of studies linking smoking to health problems, publishing a report in 1950 that showed that the risk of lung cancer was up to 50 times greater among heavy smokers compared to non-smokers

The most common cancer in women is breast cancer, which affects 20,000 women every year in Britain and causes 13,000 deaths. From 1900 to the 1960s most surgeons dealt with the disease with a radical mastectomy. This has been referred to as a 'mutilating operation', which involved removing the entire breast and much of the surrounding tissue. This was combined with radiotherapy and treatment with anti-cancer drugs. However, women are now much more likely to be given a 'lumpectomy', where only the cancerous tumour, or lump, is removed. This is a technique that was originally pioneered as far back as the 1930s by a British surgeon, Geoffrey Keynes, but which has taken some time to become acceptable and effective.

SOURCE 15

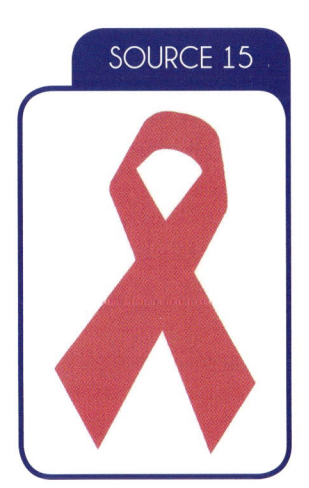

The symbol for the fight against breast cancer

The key to tackling cancer is prevention. The risk can be reduced by having regular check ups, following a healthy diet and avoiding cancer-causing activities such as smoking. Once cancer has started in the body, it can be treated through **radiotherapy**, **chemotherapy**, surgery or a combination of all three.

Today there are specialist cancer nurses like Macmillan Nurses who are fully qualified and trained to deal with patients who are suffering from cancer.

Heart disease

Many factors can cause heart disease, including unhealthy diet (fatty foods can lead to blocked arteries), smoking, stress, alcohol abuse, being overweight and various viruses. Older people are more likely to suffer from heart disease. It is the most common cause of death in the UK, causing more than one in every three deaths. Heart disease is much more common in rich countries than in poor countries.

Coronary heart disease begins when the coronary arteries (the arteries that supply blood and oxygen to the heart muscle) become narrowed by a gradual build-up of fatty materials thickening their walls – a condition called atherosclerosis. In time the artery may become so narrow that it cannot deliver enough oxygen-containing blood to the heart muscle. The resulting pain or discomfort is called angina.

If the material causing the blockage becomes unstable, it may break off and lead to a blood clot. If this blocks the coronary artery, the heart muscle is starved of blood and oxygen, and may become permanently damaged. This is known as a heart attack.

Treatment of heart disease may consist of advice about diet or exercise. A specialist Coronary Heart Disease Nurse, through a Cardiac Rehabilitation Programme provided by a Local Health Board, can provide this. Drugs to steady the pulse, to lower blood pressure or to reduce a patient's cholesterol level, can also provide treatment.

Surgery, including bypass, is also increasingly common, and electronic pacemakers can be fitted to help the heart keep up a steady beat. In extreme cases patients can be given a new heart. An increasingly common form of treatment is to carry out an angioplasty, where a 'stent' (a short tube of stainless steel mesh) is inserted permanently into an artery that has been narrowed by the build-up of fatty tissue in order to widen it. This procedure involves minimal invasive surgery.

SOURCE 16

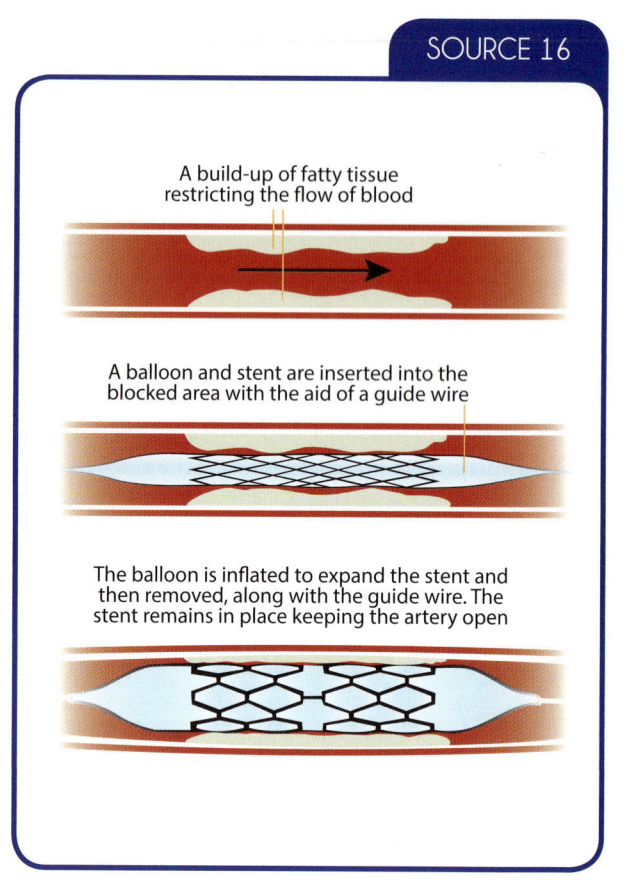

Diagram showing the procedure for inserting a stent in a narrowed artery

As heart disease is such a major killer, research into the treatment of the disease is on-going. In 2011 researchers at the University of Leicester published their findings on an injection that they claim can effectively restrict the damage caused by a heart attack or stroke. The injection has been tested on mice and other animals and has been shown to work on human blood in the laboratory. The scientists at Leicester University hope to begin human trials in 2013. If the injection is successful the £29 billion cost to the British economy in health care could be significantly reduced.

Why have cancer and heart disease become such big killers?
- Increased life expectancy – cancer and heart disease tend to be diseases of old age;
- Other diseases that have killed in the past have been conquered; cancer and heart disease are proving more difficult to cure;
- Deaths from cancer and heart disease in the past were underestimated because they were not recognised;
- Changes in lifestyle – cancer and heart disease are often 'lifestyle diseases' caused by smoking, unhealthy eating or pollution in the environment.

The HIV/AIDS threat

In 1981 a new and puzzling illness was first reported, occurring particularly in homosexual men in the USA: this illness was AIDS – Acquired Immune Deficiency Syndrome. In a sufferer a virus called HIV (Human Immunodeficiency Virus) destroys the body's immune system, reducing its defences against attack. Even a common cold can kill an AIDS sufferer. The victim doesn't die of AIDS but of other infections that the body can no longer fight. By 2000 there were an estimated 30 million people infected with AIDS and thousands of deaths a year. AIDS affects both men and women.

The worst hit area of the world is Africa, where 19 million people are currently infected with AIDS (63% of the worldwide total) and already by the year 2000 almost 8 million had died as a result. Because of AIDS, life expectancy in Uganda is the lowest in the world. Health education initiatives in African countries have tried to raise public awareness and change people's attitudes to AIDS.

At first governments reacted as if they were facing a new plague. Comparisons were made with previous sudden disasters like the medieval plague and nineteenth century cholera epidemics. However AIDS cannot be transferred by touch, or through the air. The virus is spread through the blood or other body fluids: for example, through sexual contact or by sharing hypodermic needles with an infected person. People can protect themselves from AIDS by avoiding unsafe sex and intravenous drug use.

As doctors have tracked the rapid progress of AIDS around the world they have related it to the ease of travel between different countries. It has been called a 'charter disease' because affordable charter flights between the world's major cities have helped the disease to spread. As was the case with the Black Death, isolated societies that are away from easy transport routes have been less affected by the spread of AIDS.

The AIDS threat has come as a shock to the modern world. Despite a massive amount of research there is no vaccine or magic bullet that can cure it. Azathioprine (AZT) is the principal drug that has some effect on the infection. It does help to prolong life in an infected sufferer, but it does not cure the disease.

Sufferers have often been isolated within their communities. People have looked for a scapegoat and they have pointed the finger at Africans and at gay men; some have even offered supernatural explanations for the spread of the epidemic. Other people have been more positive, encouraging a more caring and sympathetic attitude to sufferers, as shown in Source 17.

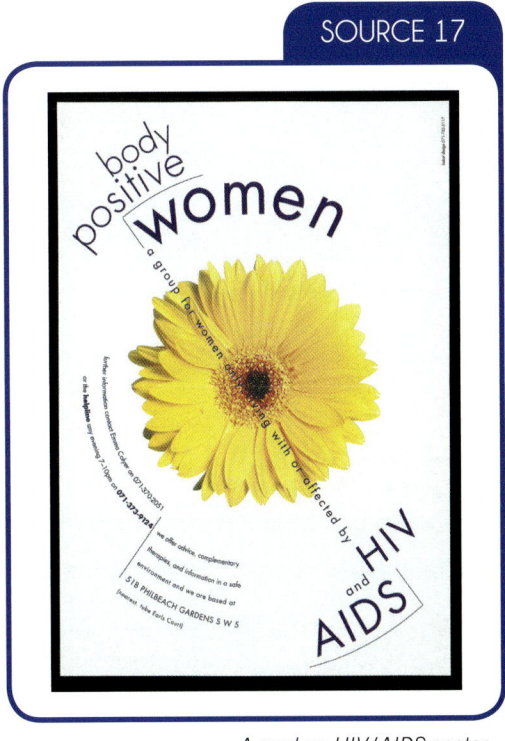

SOURCE 17

A modern HIV/AIDS poster

Keyhole and microsurgery

There are many different skills involved in surgery. Dr Christiaan Barnard had thirty people divided into two teams of specialists working with him on the first heart transplant in 1967. The specialist surgeon today continues to be supported by highly trained anaesthetists and nurses and surgery has evolved considerably, adapting techniques from the American space programme of the 1960s.

Keyhole surgery has become increasingly commonplace. In recent years, miniaturisation, fibre-optic cables and the use of computers have meant that surgeons can perform operations through very small keyhole incisions. This avoids making large incisions from which patients would take longer to recover. Keyhole surgery involves using an endoscope (an instrument to view inside the body), which can include all the tools needed to perform operations on knee joints, hernias, the gall bladder and the kidneys. Patients operated on by this method don't always need to stay in hospital overnight; it is therefore less expensive than more traditional methods of surgery.

SOURCE 18

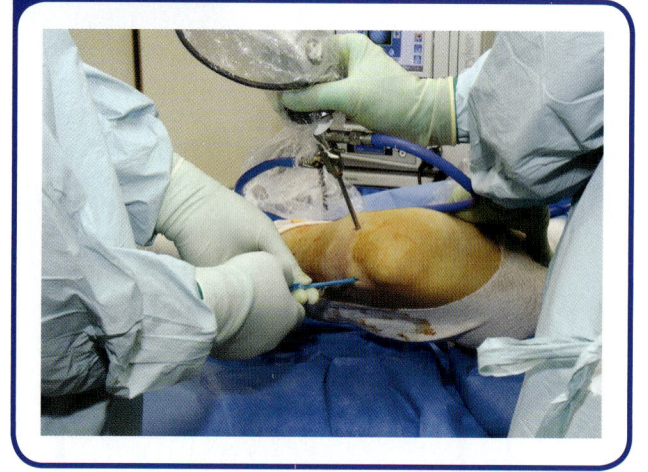

Microsurgery is also advancing very quickly. By magnifying the area on which a surgeon is working, it is possible to re-join nerves and very small blood vessels. This means that some feeling can be returned to limbs that have been damaged or even severed.

There have been considerable changes in the prevention and treatment of disease from the Middle Ages to the present day. Some of these changes have been more rapid than others. Today's modern drugs and treatments achieve a degree of success that was undreamt of in earlier centuries and further advances are likely as the twenty first century progresses.

Keyhole surgery on a knee joint

TASKS

1. Explain why and how cancer occurs.
2. Describe ways in which heart disease can be treated.
3. Do some internet research. Find 2 posters that give a positive message about AIDS. Explain your choice.
4. Explain why keyhole and microsurgery are more popular than traditional surgery.

Timeline

1. Construct a timeline of some of the major changes in the prevention and treatment of disease from the Middle Ages to the present day.
2. Which change do you think was the most significant? Explain your answer fully.

Examination practice

This section provides guidance on how to answer the synoptic question from Section B of Unit 3. The question is worth 10 marks.

Questions 4, 5 and 6 – the selection of own knowledge and the evaluation of key concepts

Have methods used to prevent and treat disease always led to improved health from the Middle Ages to the present day?

[10 marks]

You may wish to discuss the following in your answer:
- *The use of traditional treatments and remedies*
- *The development of scientific approaches to treating diseases*
- *The contributions of Simpson and Lister*
- *The development of modern surgical methods, including transplant surgery*

and any other relevant factors.

Tips on how to answer

This is an **essay question**, which is intended to cover the period you have studied. Your aim is to outline the degree of change, or lack of change, across the whole period from the Middle Ages to the present day. It is essential that you:

- Include **information from across the whole period**, although you can be selective.
- Take notice of the **information provided in the bullet points** and ensure that you cover these points, as well as additional information from your own knowledge on this topic.
- Aim to show how things have changed, or stayed the same, remembering that **the pace of change will vary across time** – it will be faster during some periods than others.
- Remember that **change did not affect all sections of society in the same way**.
- **Do not dwell too long on one time period** and aim to cover as much of the whole period as possible.
- Remember the **rules of essay writing**. Your answer will require relevant information with good quality of written communication, presented with an introduction, main paragraphs and conclusion.

Response by candidate one

Methods of preventing and treating disease have improved from the Middle Ages to the present day. In the Middle Ages traditional treatments and remedies were used, like herbal remedies and bloodletting. These were used for centuries.

The Renaissance period led to a more scientific approach to treating diseases and this led eventually to Edward Jenner discovering a vaccine for smallpox at the end of the eighteenth century. Further methods were developed in the nineteenth century with Simpson developing anaesthetics to relieve pain in operations and Lister developing antiseptics to limit infection.

Today modern surgical methods include transplant surgery. Dr Christiaan Barnard did the first heart transplant in 1967 and since then there have been many other kinds of transplants.

So, methods of preventing and treating disease have developed since the Middle Ages but they have not always led to improved health because people have died as a result of operations and are still dying from various diseases.

Examiner's comment

The answer displays a reasonable chronological grasp but with limited coverage and reference to change. The answer tends to follow the scaffold, covering the whole period of time, but there is no attempt at differentiation. The quality of written communication is sound with an attempt at introduction, main body and conclusion, and it has been presented in paragraphs. The response is just sufficient to be awarded top Level 2 for 5 marks.

Response by candidate two

Methods of preventing and treating disease have improved health a lot from the Middle Ages to the present day. However the rate of improvement has varied and some methods have not always improved health.

In the Middle Ages methods were often based on superstition and on remedies that had been used for centuries. Herbal remedies like chickweed, which was used for open sores, sometimes worked. Bloodletting, often performed by barber surgeons, was commonly used. It was an attempt to balance the humours in the body and could help to relieve pain; it could also lead to infection.

The Renaissance period from the sixteenth century was a period of discovery and of new ideas. Advances in science and anatomy began to challenge ideas like the theory of the four humours, which had been in practice for over a thousand years. The invention of the microscope in the seventeenth century meant that a more scientific approach to investigating disease was possible. This type of approach eventually led to Edward Jenner discovering a vaccine for smallpox in the 1790s. Although Jenner demonstrated that his discovery worked, there was a lot of opposition to his new method. Such negative attitudes slowed down the development of further methods, which meant that progress was slow.

In the eighteenth century attitudes were changing and surgery came to be regarded as a proper part of medicine. The scientific approaches of the previous century helped John Hunter to establish surgery as a recognised profession. He has been referred to as 'the founder of modern scientific surgery'. This was the time of the Industrial Revolution and by the early nineteenth century Britain's population was increasing rapidly and illness and disease were spreading more quickly. More operations needed to be done but there were two main problems in the operating procedure – pain and infection – that could kill patients. James Simpson addressed the problem of pain when he used chloroform as an anaesthetic in the 1840s; the problem of infection was addressed when Joseph Lister used carbolic acid as an antiseptic from 1865. These methods advanced the prevention and treatment of disease but they sometimes had a negative effect. Patients could die if too much chloroform was used, for example. Even so, these methods proved to be a turning point in surgery and the search for methods of preventing and treating disease could now advance more quickly.

By the end of the nineteenth century scientists had achieved considerable success in preventing disease. They now needed to find cures. Scientists tried to find a 'magic bullet' that could cure illnesses. Paul Ehrlich and his team developed the first 'magic bullet'. They discovered Salvarsan 606 in 1905. This was a breakthrough, but Salvarsan proved difficult to use: it could kill a patient if it was not used properly. A safer 'magic bullet' was needed that could cure many diseases without harming a patient's body. Its discovery would lead to big profits for the developing pharmaceutical industry. The answer was provided by penicillin. It was re-discovered by Alexander Fleming in 1928 and developed for mass-production by Florey and Chain in the 1940s. Penicillin proved to be the 'wonder drug' of the twentieth century. Its development was motivated by the needs of soldiers wounded in the Second World War. It has since saved millions of lives worldwide and brought in the 'antibiotic era' in the treatment of disease.

The discovery of antibiotics was an outstanding success story of the twentieth century and so was the development of transplant surgery. Heart bypass surgery was pioneered in the 1960s and the climax of this type of surgery was reached in 1967 when Dr Christiaan Barnard transplanted the first human heart. This pioneering surgery led to other forms of transplant surgery, so that kidneys, liver, the pancreas, and heart-and-lungs can now be transplanted. Transplant surgery had its initial problems in that new organs were often rejected. The invention of Cyclosporine has helped to counter this problem so that countless numbers of lives have been saved and patients' health improved due to transplant surgery.

Methods used to prevent and treat disease have evolved considerably since the Middle Ages. Each advance has benefitted from earlier discoveries. Developments were rather slow in earlier centuries but have become increasingly rapid since the nineteenth century and especially throughout the twentieth century. However, methods are still being developed to treat the various types of cancer that now exist, as well as treating the AIDS/HIV epidemic since the 1980s. Methods have generally led to improved health but there is still a need to continue to search for methods to prevent and treat new and threatening diseases.

Examiner's comment

This is a structured and well-informed account that provides an effective overview of the main developments in preventing and treating disease from the Middle Ages to the present day. There is a clear attempt to discuss the issue of change and an attempt to discuss the varying impact of change. The concluding paragraph attempts a judgement, which addresses the thrust of the question. The quality of written communication is very good and the essay is presented in paragraphs with a reasonable introduction and effective conclusion. The answer reaches Level 3 and is worthy of maximum (10) marks.

Now you have a go

Have developments in surgery always been successful from the eighteenth century to the present day?

[10 marks]

You may wish to discuss the following in your answer:
- *The work of Cheselden and the Hunter brothers*
- *The development of anaesthetics and antiseptics*
- *The contributions of McIndoe and Barnard*
- *The development of modern surgical methods, including keyhole surgery and microsurgery*

and any other relevant factors.

CHAPTER 7

HOW WERE THE SICK CARED FOR IN WALES AND ENGLAND FROM THE LATE MIDDLE AGES TO THE EIGHTEENTH CENTURY?

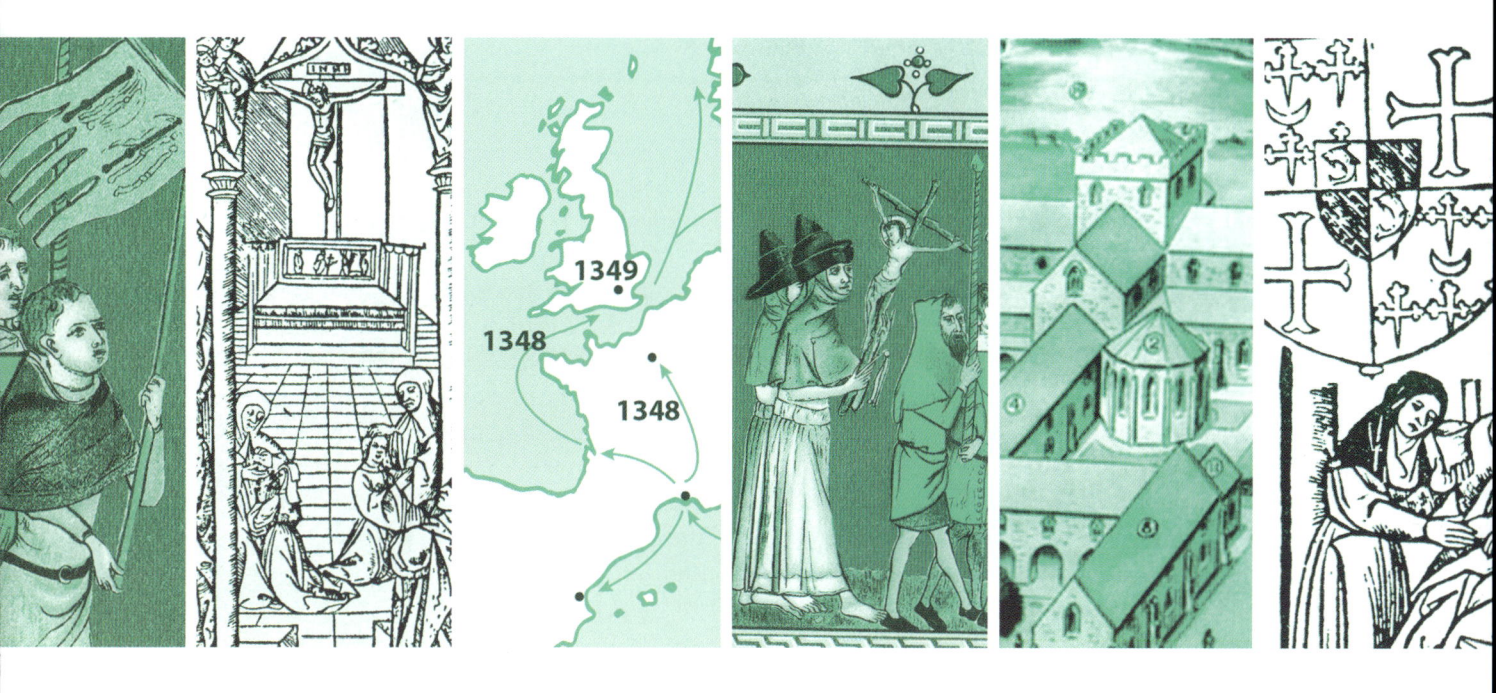

We take it for granted today that when we are ill we can visit a local doctor and have free access to hospitals. This has not always been the case and the development of these facilities and privileges has been a long process.

THE USE OF THE CHURCH AND HOSPITALS

The role of the church and medieval hospitals in caring for the sick

The Christian church taught that it was a religious duty to care for the sick. Monasteries and nunneries usually had infirmaries, which were a kind of hospital ward looked after by the inhabitants. There monks and nuns, as well as poor people or travellers who had been taken ill, could be treated. The infirmary tended to be separate from the main buildings, to avoid infection and to prevent travellers from speaking to the monks and corrupting them with worldly ideas. This was the case at Margam Abbey in south Wales and at Beaulieu Abbey in Hampshire.

In the twelfth century the Christian church started to set up hospitals, which were run by nuns and monks. They were called hospitals because they provided hospitality for visitors. Nearly 1200 of these places were created in medieval Wales and England, but they were very different from the hospitals that we have today. Most only provided food and shelter. Only a small number, known as infirmaries, provided any medical care.

- 47% housed the poor and elderly and provided no medical care;
- 31% were leper hospitals, which provided no medical care;
- 12% gave shelter to poor travellers and pilgrims;
- 10% cared for the sick.

77

SOURCE 1

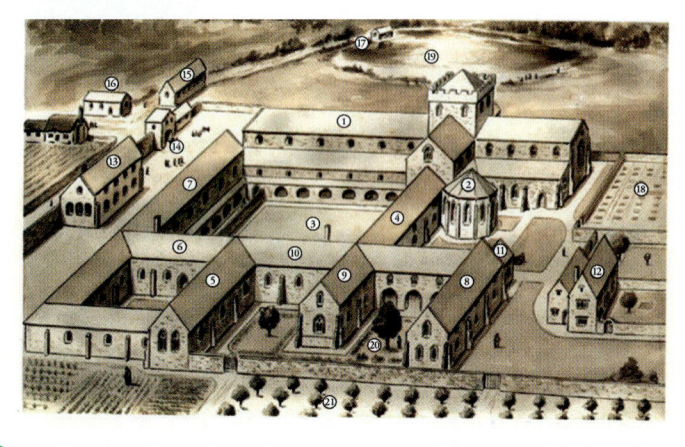

1. Church
2. Chapter House
3. Cloisters
4. Dormitory
5. Refectory
6. Kitchen
7. West Range
8. Infirmary
9. Rere Dorter
10. Warming House
11. Misericorde
12. Abbot's House
13. Guest House
14. Main Gate
15. Stables
16. Almonry
17. Mill
18. Cemetary
19. Fish Pond
20. Herbarium
21. Orchard

Margam Abbey in south Wales, showing the site of the infirmary

So, only about one in every ten medieval hospitals cared for the sick, but some of these were very large. St Leonard's Hospital in York, which was established in 1137, had room for over 200 patients and St Mary Bishopgate in London had 180 beds. Other hospitals had five or six beds.

Some medieval hospitals specialised in the care they provided. Some provided maternity care, like St Thomas' Hospital at Southwark in London; it had an eight-bed unit especially for unmarried pregnant women and also cared for old people. St Bartholomew's at Smithfield in London was a hospital for sick poor people; Christ's Hospital at Newgate cared for poor fatherless children; and Bethlehem Hospital, more commonly called 'Bedlam', was founded in 1247 for 'poor and silly persons', who were also called lunatics. The Hospital of the Blessed David in Swansea was established c.1332 for 'blind, decrepit or infirm priests and other poor men'. There were also separate leper hospitals in Britain at this time.

Pictures of the inside of a medieval hospital are rare, but Source 2 is from an engraving of the Hôtel-Dieu in Paris, which opened in 1452. This was a special hospital, as the doctors of the king of France worked there. The building measured 72 metres by 14 metres.

Hospitals had strict regulations as the following sources show.

SOURCE 3

No lepers, lunatics, or persons having the falling sickness or other contagious disease, and no pregnant women, or suckling infants, and no intolerable persons, even though they be poor and infirm, are to be admitted in the hospital. And if any such be admitted by mistake, they are to be expelled as soon as possible. And when the other poor and infirm persons have recovered they are to be let out without delay.

From the Rules of the Hospital of St John, Bridgwater, Somerset, 1219

SOURCE 2

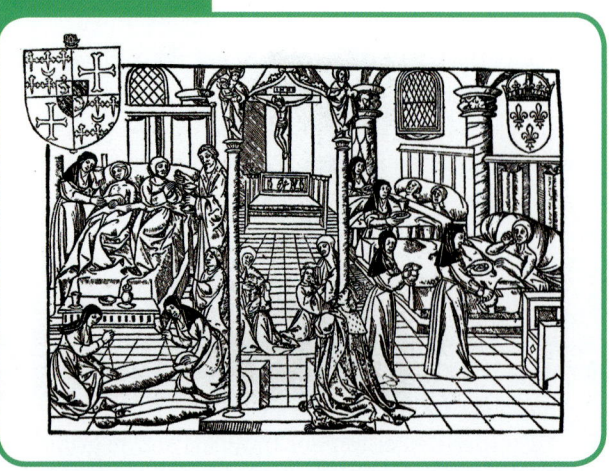

An engraving of the inside of the Hôtel-Dieu hospital in Paris

SOURCE 4

We strictly ordain ... that sick and weak people should be admitted kindly and mercifully, except for pregnant women, lepers, the wounded, cripples and the insane.

From the Rules of the Hospital of St John, Cambridge

When someone was admitted to a medieval hospital, the warden would interview them to find out about their illness. If the warden decided that the patient should be admitted, they would be led into a hall lined with beds. There were no doctors. Doctors were for kings and nobles. There would be monks in the hospital but their main job was to pray for the souls of the patients. It was usually the nuns who provided the care. They would look after the patients by bathing and feeding them, making up their beds and giving them medicines, in the form of herbal remedies.

Conditions in medieval hospitals were sometimes very bad and had not improved even into the seventeenth century, as we can see from the gruesome description of conditions given in Source 5. Nursing and the care of the sick would progress a lot in the following centuries.

SOURCE 5

'It seems likely that the approach to death ... was by way of the hospital; they were places to go in anticipation of death, not necessarily to seek a cure. ... The total dying in the Hôtel-Dieu and the other sick hospitals of Paris in the early modern period was very large. ... By the later seventeenth century, more than a quarter of all Parisians appear to have died in a hospital. Of the 21,477 recorded deaths in Paris in 1670, 4,812 ... died in the Hôtel-Dieu; another 1,105 ... died in the other hospitals. ...

The hospital [Hôtel-Dieu] was certainly a place of bad reputation, on account of its high death rate and crowded conditions. ...

The dead from the Hôtel-Dieu were taken to the burial ground fairly unceremoniously, shrouded but not coffined, on a bier, cart, or *chariot*. By the early seventeenth century the carts must have been carrying six or more, but even so, in 1656 and 1659, some *emballeurs* were reprimanded for failing to take the corpses before they began to putrefy. Nor was the shrouding adequate: Mlle de Montpensier's carriage was involved in a collision with the dead cart in 1652, and she recorded a frisson of fear at the thought of being touched by one of the hands or feet that stuck out from the cart.'

A description of the Hôtel-Dieu Hospital in Paris in the seventeenth century

TASKS

1. What does Source 1 show you about medieval infirmaries?
2. Use Sources 1 and 2 and your own knowledge to show how medieval hospitals developed.
3. Describe the role of monks and nuns in medieval hospitals.

THE IMPACT OF THE BLACK DEATH

Causes of the Black Death

The Black Death, also known as the Plague, was a terrible contagious disease that spread uncontrollably throughout Europe in the mid fourteenth century, killing many millions of people. It was carried by fleas living on infected black rats and was passed to humans through flea bites. The Black Death had started in central Asia and was carried to Europe along the trade routes from China. Trade around Europe was increasing in the fourteenth century and ships regularly sailed from the Mediterranean Sea to other parts of Europe, including Britain. Unfortunately, it was a merchant ship from France that brought the first case of the Black Death to Melcombe in Dorset in the summer of 1348.

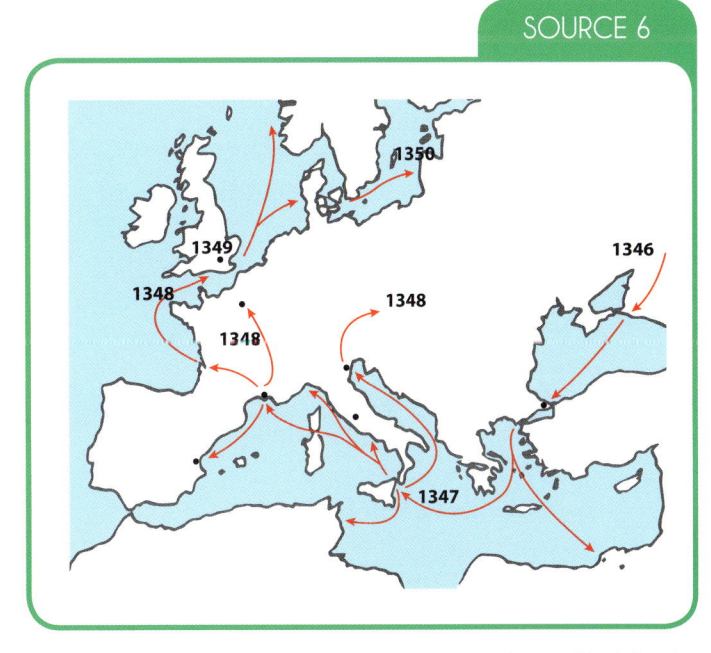

SOURCE 6

A map showing the spread of the Black Death in the mid-fourteenth century

From Melcombe, the disease spread very quickly through England, and by March 1349 it had spread along the Thames Valley to London. At one time 200 people a day were being buried in London, where huge communal graves had to be opened.

SOURCE 7

In 1348, at about the feast of the Translation of St Thomas the martyr [7 July], the cruel pestilence, hateful to all future ages, arrived from countries across the sea on the south coast of England at the port called Melcombe in Dorset. Travelling all over the south country it wretchedly killed innumerable people in Dorset, Devon and Somerset. ... Next it came to Bristol, where very few were left alive, and then travelled northwards, leaving not a city, a town, a village, or even, except rarely, a house, without killing most or all of the people there, so that over England as a whole a fifth of the men, women and children were carried to burial. As a result, there was such a shortage of people that there were hardly enough living to look after the sick and bury the dead.

An account from Eulogium Historiarum sive Temporis, *Volume III, written at Malmesbury Abbey in Wiltshire in the 1350s. Translated from Latin by Rosemary Horrox and published in* The Black Death, *1994*

By early 1349, the disease had reached Wales and over the next year it killed at least a quarter of the population. Landowner John le Strange of Whitchurch died of the Plague in August 1349. His son Fulk died eight days later, quickly followed by his brother Humphrey. The third son, John, survived, but the land and three water mills that he inherited were worthless, as the plague had also killed most of the labourers.

The Plague was, in fact, two kinds of disease:

- **Bubonic plague** – this made people suddenly feel very cold and tired. Painful swellings called buboes appeared in the armpits and the groin and black blisters appeared all over the body. The flesh rotted away and the smell was sickening. The victim's body would turn black, giving the disease its name. This was followed by high fever and severe headaches. Most victims died within three days. This form of the Black Death was spread by fleas from black rats.
- **Pneumonic plague** – this attacked the victim's lungs, causing breathing problems. Victims began to cough up blood and died more quickly than those suffering from the bubonic plague. This form of the Black Death was spread by people breathing or coughing germs onto one another.

SOURCE 8

Haint y Nodau

Nid oes drugaredd, gwedd gwiw,
gan y nod, gwenwyn ydiw.

Y nod a ddug eneidiau
y dillynion mwynion mau.
Trist y'm gwnaeth, trwy arfaeth trais,
ac unig, neur fawr gwynais.
Dwyn Ieuan wiwlan ei wedd
ymlaen y lleill naw mlynedd;
ac weithian fu'r twrn gwaethaf,
oera' swydd yn aros haf,
dihir fy nghof a'm gofeg:
dwyn Morfudd, dwyn Dafydd deg,
dwyn Ieuan, llond degan lu,
dwyn â didawddgwyn Dyddgu,
a'm gadaw, frad oerfraw fryd,
yn freiddfyw mewn afrwyddfyd.

The Pestilence

The plague has no mercy,
fine aspect, it is poison.

The plague took the lives
of my gentle darlings.
Its wilful violence made me sad
and lonely, I lamented greatly.
Handsome Ieuan was taken
nine years before the others;
and now the worst turn of all has happened,
grimmest job awaiting summer,
the memory and thought of it is painful:
Morfudd was taken, fair Dafydd was taken,
Ieuan, everyone's cheery favourite, was taken,
with an unceasing lament Dyddgu was taken,
and I was left, feeling betrayed and stunned,
barely alive in a harsh world.

An extract from a fifteenth century poem by Llywelyn Fychan, 'Haint y Nodau/The Pestilence'
(from Galar y Beirdd/Poets' Grief, *ed. Dafydd Johnston, Cardiff 1993)*

At least one fifth of the population of England was wiped out by this first occurrence of the plague and modern estimates suggest that the figure may have been as high as 40%. One Welsh writer at the time believed that half the people of Wales had died. The exact number in Wales will never be known, but the Black Death probably reached every corner of the country.

> **TASKS**
> 1. What does Source 6 show you about the spread of the Black Death?
> 2. What caused the Black Death? Describe the effects of the Black Death on a victim's body.
> 3. Study Source 8. How had the black death affected the author?

Methods of combating the Black Death

In the fourteenth century people did not know about germs but they did know that many diseases were contagious. Some town councils therefore made strict rules to keep the infection out. Travellers were not allowed to enter the town until they had waited outside its walls for at least a month. This 'quarantine' period ensured that if people had the disease they died outside the town walls, instead of bringing the infection inside.

In some European towns the first victims of the Black Death were boarded up inside their homes to die and rot along with their families. Within each family the healthy members avoided contact with the dying until they caught the disease themselves. Beggars were sometimes paid to take the dead to mass burial pits outside the town walls.

Most people simply waited, hoping that their families would survive. Some took action. The King of England and his bishops ordered churchmen to lead processions, pleading with God to end what they called 'the pestilence'. Some people made candles as tall as themselves and lit them in church as an offering to God.

A group called Flagellants whipped themselves because they thought the disease was a punishment from God for their sins. They would strip to the waist and, using whips with three or four leather thongs tipped with metal studs, whip their backs and chests until their bodies became swollen and blue, and blood ran down to the ground and splattered nearby walls. They hoped that their suffering would satisfy God's anger and that He would then get rid of the plague

Some people believed that the Black Death was due to bad air – **miasma** – and tried to avoid it by holding scented flowers to their noses. Doctors who stayed in the affected towns and cities put on gowns and hoods before making their house calls.

Other people kept their heads over buckets of dung, spending several hours every day absorbing the evil smell. They thought that the smell would somehow defeat the poison that they believed was in the air. At the same time they would take theriac, which was a cure-all medicine made from various minerals, herbs and animal flesh and blood mixed in with honey. Then following the slogan 'Fast Far Late', which meant run as fast as you can and come back as late as possible, they would leave the area!

SOURCE 9

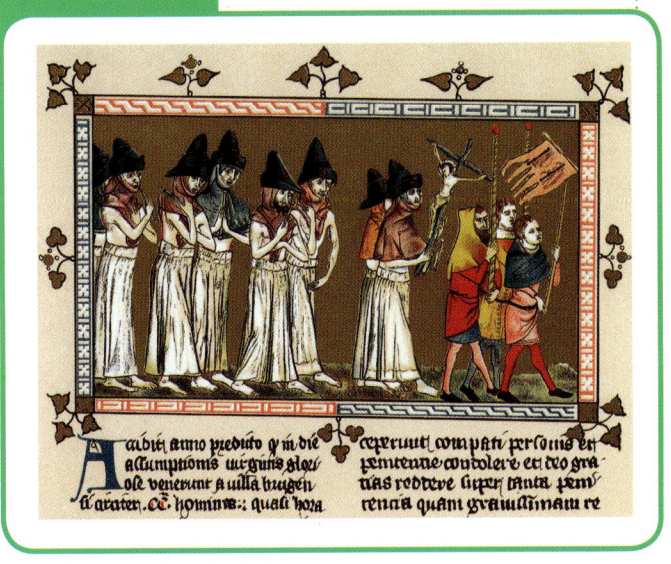

A group of flagellants in procession

WHEN A MAN IS AFFECTED WITH PLAGUE, OR BLACK POCK

Take white ox eye, (when the centre has become black) tormentil, rue, and if you like add a leaf of bay; wash these carefully, bruise with water, and administer to the patient in strong ale as hot as he can take it. Let this be done whilst the patient is in bed between sheets, and near a good fire, so that he may perspire freely. By God's help, the eruption will be transferred to the sheets.

The Physicians of Myddvai/Meddygon Myddfai, *John Pughe, 1861, p. 436*

People were also advised to clean their homes thoroughly, burn brushwood indoors and then disinfect the house with herbs. Some also burned the clothes of victims of the Black Death in order to stop the spread of the infection.

The Black Death even affected the small market town of Builth Wells in mid Wales. When the disease reached there in about 1350 the townspeople were quarantined. People from the sourrounding countryside left provisions for the inhabitants on the banks of a small brook at the edge of the town. The townspeople threw money into the brook to pay for these provisions. The water would cleanse the money, stopping the infection spreading. As a result the brook became known as 'Nant yr Arian' (Money Brook).

SOURCE 10

The Black Death of 1349 is a turning-point ... It initiated a long period in which the basic material forces working on society were different from what they had been in the central Middle Ages ... The first plague of 1349 was unmatched in its ferocity but it began a long period, ending only with the Great Plague of London in 1665, in which pestilence frequently recurred.

Historian George Holmes, writing in The Later Middle Ages, 1272-1485, *1962*

Doctors had done very little to help during this terrible time. They had not learned from the impact of the Black Death and the complex link between disease and germs was still not understood. Two inventions were needed before the link would be recognised: the printing press at the end of the fifteenth century and the microscope in the seventeenth century. However the Black Death had shown that there was a connection between disease and dirt. Despite this, towns and cities remained a breeding ground for infection and vermin and this is why many more outbreaks of the plague occurred over the next three hundred years.

The huge death toll resulting from the Black Death meant that there were not enough people left to work the land in the countryside. Detailed study has shown that in the Llanrhystud area of Ceredigion in west Wales, only seven out of 104 workers survived the Black Death. As there were fewer workers, they were able to demand higher wages, shorter hours and better working conditions. However, some workers had to work much harder in order to do the work of those who had died.

By the end of 1351 the plague had spread over all of Europe and scarcely a village was left untouched. The smell of death was everywhere, but the horror was coming to an end. However, the plague visited Wales and England many more times, with the last outbreak in Wales occurring in Haverfordwest in 1652, killing about 300 of the population of 2,500 in six months. The last recorded major outbreak in Britain was the Great Plague of London in 1665.

TASKS

1. What does Source 9 show you about how people viewed the Black Death?
2. Describe some methods of combating the Black Death.
3. Why was the Black Death a turning point in history?

Examination practice

This section provides extra guidance on how to answer Question 1(a), 2(a) and 3(a) from Unit 3. It is a source comprehension question, which is worth 2 marks.

Question 1(a), 2(a), 3(a) – comprehension of a source

(The source could be a photograph, a cartoon, a map, a graph or a written account.)

What does Source A tell you about medieval hospitals?

[2 marks]

SOURCE A

Some medieval hospitals specialised in the care they provided. Some provided maternity care, like St Thomas' Hospital at Southwark in London … St Bartholomew's at Smithfield … was a hospital for sick poor people; Christ's Hospital at Newgate cared for poor fatherless children; and Bethlehem Hospital, more commonly called 'Bedlam', was founded in 1247 for … lunatics. The Hospital of the Blessed David in Swansea was established c.1332 for 'blind, decrepit or infirm priests and poor men'.

A description of the specialism of some medieval hospitals

Tips on how to answer

This is an inference question involving the comprehension of a source.

- You are asked to **extract relevant information** from the source.
- You must also **make use of the statement written below the source**, which is intended to provide you with additional information.
- You must only **comment on the information that you can extract** from the source and what is written immediately below it. **Do not** bring in additional factual knowledge, as this will not score you marks.
- To obtain maximum marks you will need to pick out at least **two relevant points**.

Response by candidate

Source A tells us that some medieval hospitals specialised in the care that they offered. Some offered maternity care, some cared for sick poor people, others cared for poor fatherless children, some cared for lunatics, and others for blind, infirm men. These hospitals were in London and Swansea and the source tells us that Bedlam was founded in the thirteenth century, which is the medieval period.

Examiner's comment

The candidate has picked valid points from both the source and the statement written below it. The answer shows an understanding of the care offered by medieval hospitals and has fitted in the answer to the correct time frame. This is a developed answer worthy of maximum (2) marks.

Now you have a go

What does Source B tell you about the Black Death?

[2 marks]

SOURCE B

[The Black Death] was carried by fleas living on infected black rats and was passed to humans through flea bites. The Black Death had started in central Asia and was carried to Europe along the trade routes from China. ... Unfortunately, it was a merchant ship from France that brought the first case of the Black Death to Melcombe in Dorset in the summer of 1348. ...

By early 1349, the disease had reached Wales and over the next year it killed at least a quarter of the population.

A description of the Black Death in Britain

CHAPTER 8

WHAT WERE THE MAIN ADVANCES IN PUBLIC HEALTH AND PATIENT CARE IN WALES AND ENGLAND IN THE NINETEENTH CENTURY?

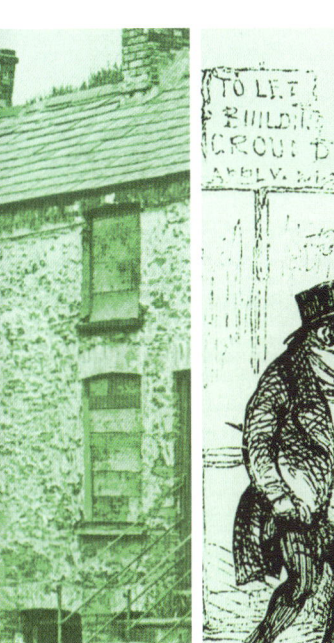

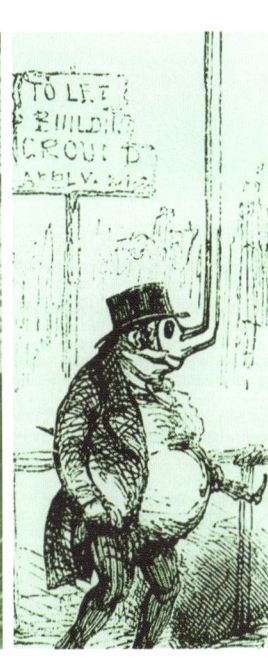

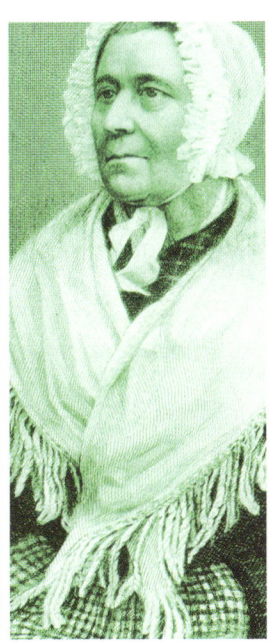

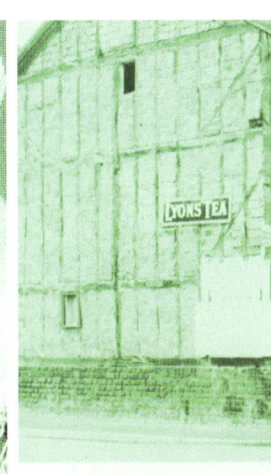

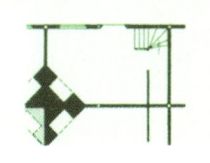

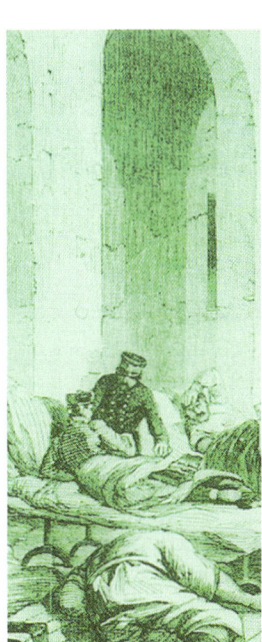

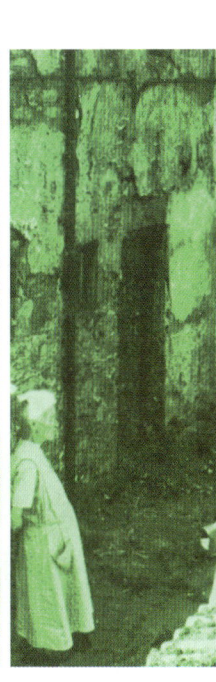

The nineteenth century witnessed important advances both in public health and in patient care in Wales and England. Attitudes to the provision of both services changed radically. Wales and England gradually became healthier places in which to live.

THE IMPACT OF INDUSTRIALISATION

Towns in the Middle Ages had been very dirty. The streets often had open sewers running down the middle. These sewers became clogged with rubbish and excrement thrown from windows. Pigs, dogs and rats often roamed freely. Large towns like London tried to clean up the streets, but not very often. These dirty conditions had contributed to the spread of the Black Death in the fourteenth century and to the outbreaks of plague in following centuries. However, no-one was interested in dealing with the problems.

This situation continued into the nineteenth century. Parish officials and central government at the beginning of the nineteenth century were still not interested in public health. It was not their concern and it was expensive. They believed in *laissez faire* or 'leave alone' and this is what they thought the local authorities and central government should do – leave things alone and not interfere.

However, conditions in the towns were now very different as industry developed in Britain in the second half of the eighteenth century. The crowded towns that grew up as a result of industrialisation meant that there had to be a different attitude to public health.

Public health problems in industrial towns

With the Industrial Revolution the growth of factories was rapid. Some small villages became manufacturing towns almost overnight. The earliest and most dramatic changes happened in Lancashire. Here, Manchester became one of the world's greatest industrial and commercial centres. Its population rose from 10,000 in 1700 to 95,000 in 1801, making it the largest town in Britain outside London. Its rapid growth was due to the development of steam-powered machinery. In 1786 there was just one steam-powered textile factory in Manchester; by 1801 there were 50. By 1821 Manchester's population had risen to 150,000 and by 1851 to 240,000. At the same time, the populations of Glasgow, Birmingham and Liverpool had also risen to over 100,000.

The Industrial Revolution also affected Wales, especially in the south. There were already small copper smelting works in Swansea in 1720, but over the next 150 years many more were opened along the Tawe Valley, as well as coal mines and works to process zinc and tin. As a result, the population grew from around 2,000 in the late 17th century to over 10,000 by 1841. In Merthyr Tydfil between 1759 and 1784, four ironworks were opened and the town was connected by rail to several ports. The population grew from just under 8,000 in 1801 to over 46,000 in 1851. Ironworks were also established in Blaenavon in 1788, and steel making and coal mining soon followed, causing the population to grow to over 20,000 at one time, before the ironworks were closed in 1900.

SOURCE 1

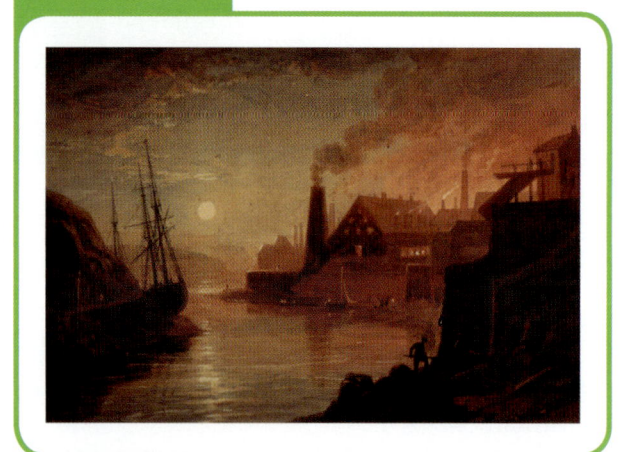

Copperworks and the river Tawe, Swansea, by Henri Gastineau, 1830

In the rush to put up factories and rows of workers' dwellings in these fast growing industrial towns, many important services were neglected. There were hardly any building regulations and there were no sanitary inspectors at this time. As a result, the rapidly built houses were often damp, streets were unpaved and full of holes, and proper sewers were almost unheard of. There was no collection of refuse, and drinking water was so scarce that it often had to be bought from street traders.

Not surprisingly in these conditions, diseases such as cholera and typhoid frequently spread through the newly created industrial towns. As soon as new houses were built, the overflowing population reduced them to crowded, disease-ridden slums.

Seeing the chance to make quick profits, builders put up as many houses as space would permit, using material of the poorest quality. Rows of dwellings were often built back-to-back, which meant that through ventilation was impossible and parts of the houses received no direct sunlight. Such houses were very unhealthy.

SOURCE 2

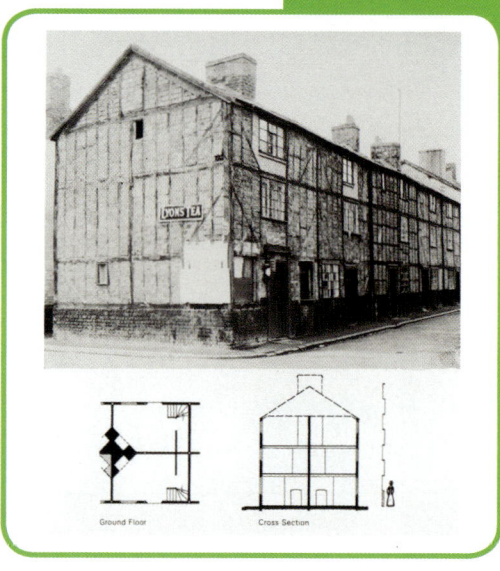

Back-to-back housing, Ladywell Street, Newtown

In Liverpool and Manchester there were large **tenement** houses. These tended to be overcrowded with several large families in each. There were even waterlogged cellars, which were rented out as separate dwellings.

SOURCE 3

The greatest portion of these districts … are of very recent origin; and … are untraversed by common sewers. The houses are ill soughed, often ill ventilated, unprovided with privies, and in consequence, the streets which are narrow, unpaved, and worn into deep ruts, become the common receptables of mud, refuse, and disgusting ordure. …
In Parliament-street there is only one privy for three hundred and eighty inhabitants, which is placed in a narrow passage, whence its effluvia infest the adjacent houses, and must prove a most fertile source of disease.

From The Moral and Physical Condition of the Working Classes Employed in the Cotton Manufacture in Manchester *by James Phillips Kay, M.D., Manchester, 1832, pp. 13, 23*

An account of one district in Newcastle in 1842 told how blood from several slaughter houses ran into a gutter. It also noted the filthy state of the shared privies (toilets) used by people living in small houses and single rooms. As no-one wanted to clean them, when the toilets got too dirty people would just use the footpath.

The availability of drinking water was a frequent problem. A statement to a health inspector at Dudley in the West Midlands in 1851 described how people often had to steal water or drink from a well that often had cats and dogs in it.

Jacob's Island in the East End of London was surrounded by a sewage-filled ditch. Wooden shacks on the banks of the ditch were used as privies that emptied their contents into the water, which was then used for drinking.

Henry Mayhew wrote a survey on the poor people in London. When he visited Jacob's Island he recorded:

SOURCE 4

As we passed along the reeking banks of the sewer the sun shone upon a narrow slip of the water. In the bright light it appeared the colour of strong green tea, and positively looked as solid as black marble in the shadow ... we saw drains and sewers emptying their filthy contents into it; we saw a whole tier of doorless privies in the open road, common to men and women, built over it; we heard bucket after bucket of filth splash into it ... And yet, as we stood ... we saw a little child, from one of the galleries opposite, lower a tin can with a rope to fill a large bucket that stood beside her.

From London Labour and the London Poor, *2012*

In such horrific conditions cholera, which was spread when drinking water was contaminated by the drains, appeared in the industrial towns with dire consequences in the first half of the nineteenth century.

TASKS

1. Describe the *laissez faire* attitude to public health.
2. What does Source 1 show you about conditions in industrial towns?
3. Use Source 2 to explain why back-to-back housing was unhealthy.
4. Use Sources 3 and 4 to explain why diseases were so common at these locations.

The effect of industrial developments in Wales

The fastest growing town in Wales during the Industrial Revolution was the iron-producing town of Merthyr Tydfil. In 1723 the traveller and writer Daniel Defoe visited the town during his tour through Britain. He recorded that the district around Merthyr Tydfil was a "most agreeable vale opening to the south with a pleasant river running through it called the Taafe".

However, when two members of a family of London lawyers visited the area in 1819, their impression was very different.

SOURCE 5

about five miles from Merthyr, we saw in the atmosphere a faint glimmering redness appearing at intervals; as we advanced it became more fixed with occasional deeper flashes, and we were now convinced that it was the glare from the numerous furnaces in the neighbourhood of the Town. After walking a mile or two farther, we could discover the flames from some of the chimnies, which illumined the atmosphere in that quarter, while behind every thing was in utter darkness heightened by a thick wet fog. The road was miserably bad and dirty, but the novelty and grandeur of the sight prevented our thinking of any inconveniences or fatigue; we could now see the men moving about among the blazing fires, and hear the noise of huge hammers, clanking of chains, whiz of wheels, blast of bellows, with the deep roaring of the fires, which soon increased to a stunnig degree. The effect was almost terrific when contrasted to the pitchy darkness of the night.

William and Sampson Sandys, writing in Walk through South-Wales in October 1819, *pp. 30-31*

In fact the two London lawyers had encountered the Penydarren Ironworks. This was one of four major ironworks in the town that had made Merthyr Tydfil not only Wales' first completely industrial town, but also the largest town in Wales' history up to that time. Typically of the newly developed industrial towns at this time, Merthyr Tydfil had grown very rapidly from a population of 7,705 in 1801 to 46,378 by 1851.

SOURCE 6

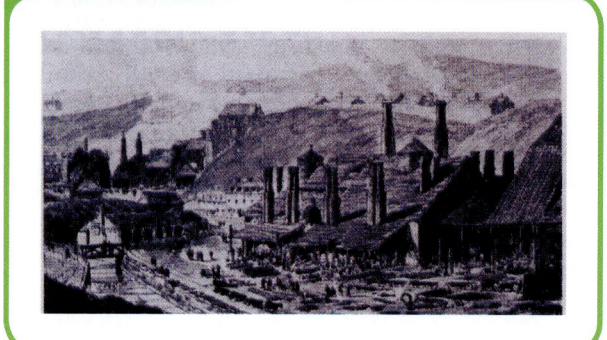

Penydarren Ironworks, 1813, showing workers' housing left of centre

To supply the demand for housing in this rapidly growing industrial town, as elsewhere in industrial Britain, houses were built as quickly and cheaply as possible. They were crammed together in the areas around the new works. Local sandstone was mainly used for building, as it was cheap and easily available. However sandstone is very absorbent and it let in water, making the houses very damp. A visitor to Merthyr Tydfil in the very early nineteenth century described the way houses were developing in the town, as Source 7 shows.

SOURCE 7

The first houses that were built were only very small and simple cottages for furnace-men, forge-men, miners, and such tradesmen as were necessary to construct the required buildings ... These cottages were most of them built in scattered confusion, without any order or plan. As the works increased, more cottages were wanted, and erected in the spaces between those that had been previously built

B. H. Malkin, writing in The Scenery, Antiquities and Biography of South Wales, from Materials Collected during Two Excursions in the Year 1803, *Vol. 1 (1807), p. 269*

The enclosed spaces between houses were called courts and, as Source 8 shows, they were very confined. People lived in these courts well into the twentieth century.

SOURCE 8

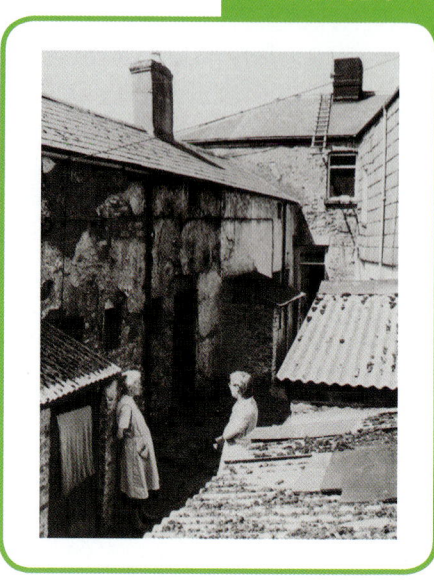

Baili Glas Court at Twyn-yr-Odyn, Merthyr Tydfil

The houses that were packed into these courts were very small and unhealthy.

SOURCE 9

A large number of these cottages consist of only two rooms, the upper being the sleeping apartment for the family, and usually ill-ventilated. Mr Davies, superintendent of the Merthyr police, states, that in these two-roomed houses, occupied by workmen, there are generally three beds in the sleeping apartment, containing five or six persons. These cottages are often very small, 8 feet by 10 feet and 8 feet by 12 feet, being not uncommon.

From 'Report on the Sanatory Condition of Merthyr Tydfil, Glamorganshire' by Sir Henry T. De La Beche in Second Report of the Commissioners for Inquiring into the State of Large Towns and Populous Districts. With Appendix – Part I. (1845), p. 146

The above report was written by the Royal Commission on the Health of Towns, appointed by the government in 1843. This report showed that the government was at last aware of the appalling conditions in which some working people were living and becoming concerned with public health issues. Sir Henry T. De La Beche further reported that the worst part of the town of Merthyr Tydfil was an area known as 'The Cellars', where 1500 people lived in cramped and unhealthy conditions.

SOURCE 10

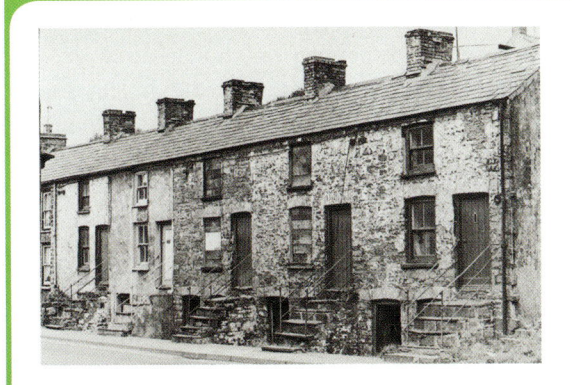

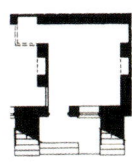

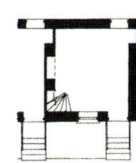

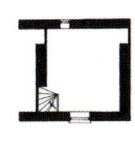

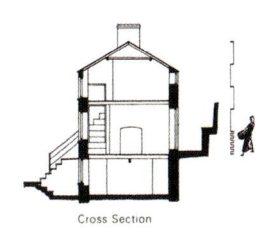

Plymouth Street, Merthyr Tydfil, built in the 1840s. The upper houses had two rooms each; the basements were separate single room dwellings called the 'cellars', as we can see in the cross-section

Sir Henry T. De La Beche reported of these cellar dwellings in the 1845 report:

"they are not cellars, but a collection of small houses of two stories, situated in a depression between a line of road and a cinder heap … The space between these houses is generally very limited; and an open, stinking, and nearly stagnant gutter, into which the house refuse is, as usual, flung, moves slowly before the doors. It is a labyrinth of miserable tenements and filth"

The difficulties of obtaining water in Merthyr Tydfil were a particular problem, as people had to que for it at waterspouts in the street. Sometimes women would queue for up to ten hours at a time for their turn and then some would have to leave without any water at all.

Without proper sanitation or a clean and regular water supply, the filthy conditions in the poorest part of Merthyr Tydfil led to waves of cholera and typhoid epidemics sweeping through the town in the first half of the nineteenth century.

TASKS

1. Describe the ways in which Merthyr Tydfil changed in the early nineteenth century.
2. Describe the role of Sir Henry T. De La Beche in Merthyr Tydfil in 1844.
3. Explain why water was a particular problem in Merthyr Tydfil.

Cholera

1832, 1849, 1854 and 1866 have been referred to as 'the four great cholera years in Wales'. In the summer months of each of those years, cholera caused hundreds of deaths.

In north Wales, cholera reached Flint early in May 1832. The disease then spread to Bagillt and on to Holywell. By the end of July there had been 49 deaths in Holywell and the disease had spread widely in north Wales – to Abergele, Llanrwst and Llandrillo. At Denbigh, 34 people died in less than a month. Cholera then spread to other parts of the country.

Deaths in selected Welsh towns from the 1832 cholera epidemic	
Newport	13
Abergavenny	2
Merthyr Tydfil	160
Swansea	152
Haverfordwest	16
Denbigh	47
Caernarvon	30
Flint	18
Newtown	17

Data from A History of Epidemics in Britain by Charles Creighton, 1894, p. 822

The first case of cholera in the 1849 epidemic occurred in Cardiff, with the death rate rising to 135 in June. The disease then spread to Newport. Aberystwyth also suffered an outbreak. However, Merthyr Tydfil suffered the greatest losses, with a peak of 349 deaths in June.

SOURCE 11

> I am sorry to say that the accounts of the cholera at Dowlais are fearfully bad. They are beyond anything I could have imagined, sometimes upwards of twenty people dying in one day, and eight men constantly employed in making coffins. Poor Miss Diddams, one of our Infant School – Mistresses, is dead. One of the medical assistants sent down from London is dying, and the whole place seems in a most lamentable state. I am greatly grieved at the conditions of my poor home

From Lady Charlotte Guest. Extracts from her journal 1833-1852, *31 July 1849, p. 230. Lady Charlotte was the wife of the owner of the Dowlais Ironworks*

A further 539 people died in the Merthyr district in July 1849. There were no hospital facilities, but the ironmaster, J. J. Guest, opened a refuge for the healthy and a night dispensary for cholera cases, where free medicines could be obtained. Cholera then spread in south Wales to Neath, Swansea, Llanelli and Carmarthen.

In north Wales, Holywell and Flint again suffered. The disease then spread to the villages of Northop and Halkyn. Two cholera deaths occurred in the Wrexham Workhouse but the town itself escaped the worst of the disease. In mid Wales, Welshpool suffered a severe epidemic and there were 34 deaths in a crowded slum area of the town.

Cholera Deaths in some Welsh Towns in 1849			
Newport	209	Ystradgynlais	107
Pontypool	61	Llanelly District	45
Tredegar	203	Swansea	262
Aberystwyth	223	Carmarthen	102
Crickhowell	95	Welshpool	34
Cardiff	396	Newtown	6
Neath	245	Holywell	46
Margam	241	Flint	35
Maesteg	33	Caernarvon	16
Bridgend	50	Holyhead	42
Merthyr District	1682	Amlwch	22

Monthly Deaths May-November in the Registrar Districts of Cardiff, Merthyr Tydfil and Neath, 1849							
	May	June	July	August	Sept	Oct	Nov
Cardiff	39	135	69	91	55	3	1
Merthyr Tydfil	16	349	539	548	190	37	3
Neath	5	80	296	260	84	10	0

From 'Cholera in Wales' by G. Penrhyn Jones in The National Library of Wales Journal, *Summer 1958*

There were two further major cholera epidemics in Wales in 1854 and in 1866 and the government was becoming increasingly concerned about the bad living conditions in the industrial towns. An 'Enquiry into Merthyr Tydfil' had been ordered in 1850, which highlighted the water supply problems in the town.

However, it was the cholera epidemics of 1832 and 1849 that were the turning points; they emphasized the problem of public health in the industrial towns of Wales, showing that improvements were needed urgently.

> **TASKS**
>
> 1. What does the list of deaths from the 1832 epidemic tell you about cholera in Wales?
> 2. Look at the list of deaths from the 1849 epidemic. Why do you think that there were more deaths in south Wales than in the north?
> 3. What does the list of monthly deaths in 1849 tell you about the cholera epidemic?
> 4. Explain why the 1832 and 1849 cholera epidemics were turning points.

PUBLIC HEALTH IMPROVEMENTS

Cholera was new to Britain in the nineteenth century. The first recorded victim of cholera in Britain was William Sproat, who died in October 1831 in the filthy slums near Sunderland docks in north east England. The disease had long been known in India but now it had spread to other parts of the world. It took several British doctors with experience in India to recognise this new killer.

By 1832 cholera had spread to most towns in Britain. The newly developed industrial towns were especially at risk. In the 1831-32 epidemic, at least 32,000 deaths were officially recorded, but many more went unrecorded. The limited action taken to counter the epidemic was local and disorganized.

SOURCE 12

I was called, on Sunday, the 23rd of October, to visit William Sproat, a **keelman**, living near the Long Bank, in the parish of Sunderland …
    I found him evidently sinking; pulse almost imperceptible [unnoticeable], and extremities [hands and feet] cold, skin dry, eyes sunk, lips blue, features shrunk, he spoke in whispers, violent vomiting and purging, cramps of the calves of the legs, and complete prostration [loss] of strength. … the urine was suppressed. … On Tuesday, October 25th, … [I] ordered … brandy … and opium … On Wednesday morning, October the 26th, he was much weaker; the pulse scarcely beating under the fingers, … lips dark blue, as well as the skin of the lower extremities, the nails were livid [black]; he was comatose [unconscious]; … at twelve o'clock at noon he died.

Extract from the report of Mr Holmes, a surgeon, on the death of William Sproat, 26 October 1831, as recorded in Hyperanthraxis; or, The Cholera of Sunderland by W. Reid Clanny, 1832, pp.20, 23-25

Cholera terrified people because of the speed at which it spread, the fact that it affected rich and poor alike and the suffering that it caused its victims. They had no idea at the time that it was transmitted through contaminated water. Germs from the excreta of infected people were carried from the privies to the water supply. Once contaminated, anyone using that supply could pick up the cholera germs. Some people believed that the disease was a punishment from God; some believed it was spread by touch; others still believed in the **miasma** theory (see Chapter 3). There was a lack of understanding and people were very worried.

The work of Edwin Chadwick

Edwin Chadwick (1800-90) was born near Manchester and was probably one of the greatest reformers of his age. He had been appointed as a Poor Law Commissioner in 1832 and his report of 1833 formed the basis for the Poor Law of 1834. In his work as Poor Law Commissioner, Chadwick had become aware of the dreadful living conditions in the industrial towns. He decided to lead a campaign to improve public health and to wipe out dreaded diseases like cholera. Chadwick himself believed in the miasma theory of disease.

SOURCE 13

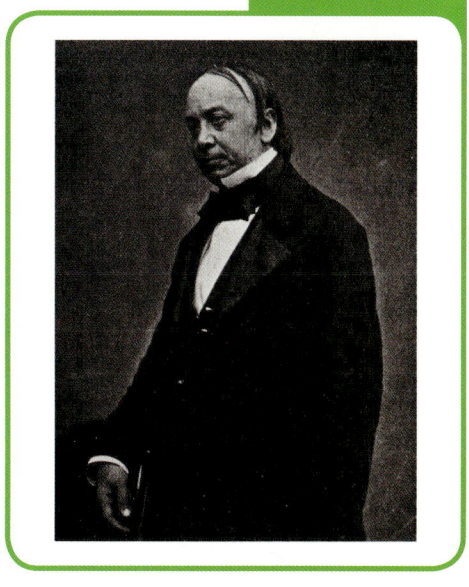

Edwin Chadwick, 1800-1890

Chadwick wanted to find out exactly what living conditions were like for working people. He was convinced that there was a link between poor health and bad living conditions. In 1838 he appointed three doctors – Doctors Kay, Arnott and Southwood Smith – to investigate housing conditions in East London. The registration of births, marriages and deaths had been made compulsory in 1836 and the resulting records helped considerably with the work. The evidence produced by these three doctors revealed for the first time to the middle-classes and to the government the terrible conditions in which most working people lived.

The government was impressed by Chadwick's investigation. They set up a Royal Commission in 1839 to carry out a nationwide survey of living conditions for working people. Chadwick was appointed head of this Commission.

In 1842 Chadwick published his findings in the 'Report from the Poor Law Commissioners on an Inquiry into the Sanitary Conditions of the Labouring Population of Great Britain'. It was the most detailed examination of the problem up to that time. The report caused great controversy. Chadwick had learned from his experience with earlier official reports that shock tactics were an effective way of getting Parliament to act. So he filled his report with graphic descriptions of the illnesses that were endured by working people. The report sold 20,000 copies and a further 10,000 were given away. These were very large numbers for the time.

SOURCE 14

'First, as to the extent and operation of the evils which are the subject of the inquiry:-

That the various forms of epidemic, endemic, and other disease caused, or aggravated, or propagated chiefly amongst the labouring classes by atmospheric impurities produced by decomposing animal and vegetable substances, by damp and filth, and close and overcrowded dwellings prevail amongst the population in every part of the kingdom, whether dwelling in separate houses, in rural villages, in small towns, in the larger towns – as they have been found to prevail in the lowest districts of the metropolis.

That such disease, wherever its attacks are frequent, is always found in connexion with the physical circumstances above specified, and that where those circumstances are removed by drainage, proper cleansing, better ventilation, and other means of diminishing atmospheric impurity, the frequency and intensity of such disease is abated; and where the removal of the noxious agencies appears to be complete, such disease almost entirely disappears.

That high prosperity in respect to employment and wages, and various and abundant food, have afforded to the labouring classes no exemptions from attacks of epidemic disease, which have been as frequent and as fatal in periods of commercial and manufacturing prosperity as in any others.

That the formation of all habits of cleanliness is obstructed by defective supplies of water.'

From 'Report from the Poor Law Commissioners on an Inquiry into the Sanitary Conditions of the Labouring Population of Great Britain', Parliamentary Papers (1842), p. 369

Chadwick's belief in the miasma theory of disease is evident from his report. He had highlighted many of the deficiencies in working people's living conditions referred to earlier in this chapter. His report quoted hundreds of examples to support his conclusions. One of the most famous pieces of evidence was his comparison of age of death in the countryside with age of death in towns, as shown in Source 15.

SOURCE 15

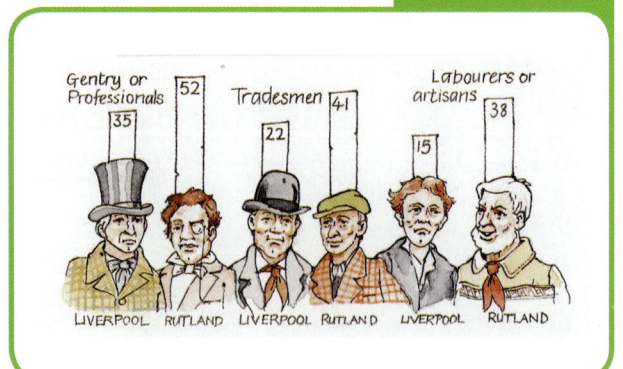

Diagram showing the average age of death in Liverpool (an urban area) and Rutland (a rural area) in 1840

Gentry or Professionals: Liverpool 35, Rutland 52
Tradesmen: Liverpool 22, Rutland 41
Labourers or artisans: Liverpool 15, Rutland 38

Chadwick's Report highlighted four main issues:
- Disease killed more citizens than any wars;
- Parliament should pass and enforce laws to make drainage and sanitation effective;

- These measures should be funded from local rates and small increases in rents;
- Bad conditions led to immoral behaviour, not the other way around.

Chadwick recommended that local authorities should become responsible for improving drainage, removing refuse from dwellings and streets, and improving water supplies. He further recommended that a district medical officer should be appointed, with responsibility for introducing sanitary improvements. Chadwick also recommended that there should be a national body to organize sanitary improvements, as huge engineering schemes would be required to improve drainage and sewerage nationwide.

Edwin Chadwick was well aware of the need for economy and argued that the expense of sanitary improvements would be offset by reduced costs of treating illness and disease. He said that if the government followed his suggestions, the effect would be dramatic and would lead to an increase of at least 13 years in the life expectancy of the labouring classes.

TASKS

1. How significant was the death of William Sproat?
2. Rewrite the first paragraph of Source 14 in your own words.
3. Why was Chadwick's report of 1842 important for public health reform?
4. What does Source 15 tell you about life expectancy in the mid ninetenth century?

Victorian health legislation

Despite its impact, Chadwick's report did not lead to immediate action. The government did little in the next few years to improve public health, but they did appoint another Royal Commission in 1843. This was the 'Health of Towns Commission', which, as we have seen, reported on Merthyr Tydfil through Sir Henry T. De La Beche. The Commission interviewed doctors, Poor Law officials, engineers and architects. Chadwick was not officially involved in the Commission, but he was the guiding force. He chose the witnesses and he supervised the inspections and the interviews.

SOURCE 16

My vacation has been absorbed in visiting with Mr Smith & Dr Playfair the worst parts of some of our worst towns. Dr Playfair has been knocked up by it and has been seriously ill. Mr Smith has had a little dysentery. Sir Henry De La Beche was obliged at Bristol to stand at the end of alleys and vomit whilst Dr Playfair was investigating overflowing privies. Sir Henry was obliged to give it up.

Part of a letter by Edwin Chadwick to Major George Graham, 7 December 1843

The Commission published its report in 1844 and this led to:
- The formation of the Health of Towns Association in 1844;
- The introduction of a Public Health Bill to Parliament. However, opponents of public health reform, who became known as the 'Dirty Party', defeated this;
- In 1847 Liverpool appointed a Medical Officer of Health and Manchester and Glasgow followed this example.

In 1848 another cholera epidemic occurred in Britain. Once again the killer disease helped to advance the public health movement. With cholera raging, the Dirty Party dropped their opposition to reform and the Public Health Act was passed.

The Public Health Act, 1848

- A general Board of Health was set up, with Lord Shaftesbury and Edwin Chadwick as members.
- Any town could set up a board of health if 10% of the ratepayers were in agreement. If the death rate reached 23 in one thousand, a town had to have a board of health.
- Local boards had the power to: appoint officials; connect older houses to sewers; make sure new houses had drainage; supply water or supervise existing water companies; provide public parks; inspect slaughter houses; collect a local rate to pay for the measures.

These features of the 1848 Act would address the main public health problems suffered in Britain at this time and Chadwick set to work with enthusiasm. The Board of Health tried to work with local boards wherever possible. With the cholera epidemic of 1848-49 killing over 50,000 people there was considerable interest in public health reform. The construction of a network of sewers was one of the greatest achievements of the Board of Health. The Board recommended glazed earthenware pipes for new sewerage systems. These were more hygienic than brick and were also cheaper. Between 1848 and 1856, 2,500 miles of new sewerage pipes were laid. Chadwick's efforts were at last leading to considerable success. Public health issues were now being kept in the public eye as the following two sources show.

SOURCE 18

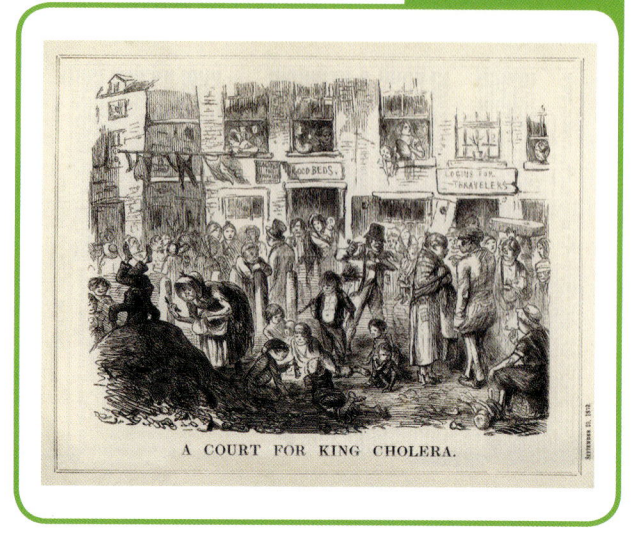

A cartoon illustrating the many threats to health in a crowded urban environment

SOURCE 17

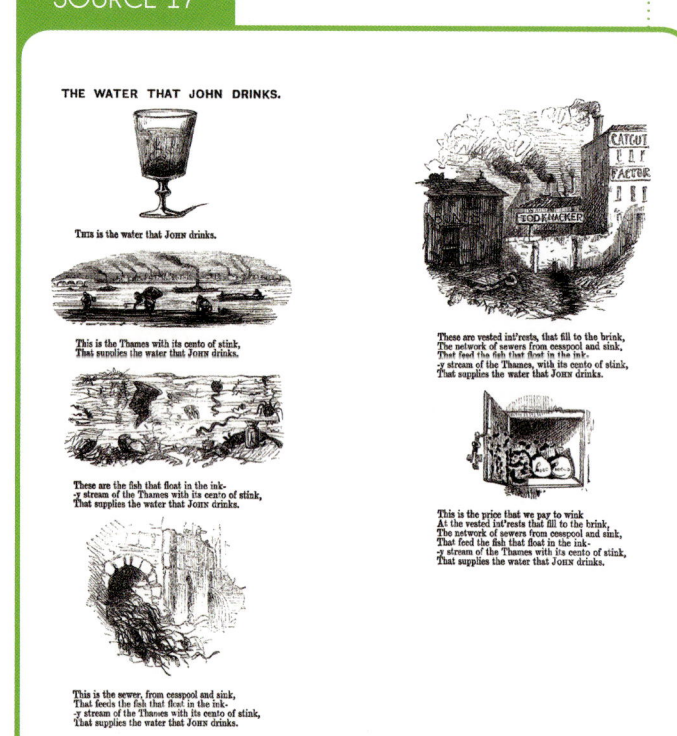

A cartoon from Punch *magazine, highlighting the problems of contaminated drinking water, October 1849*

Unfortunately, the Public Health Act of 1848 was limited. It was a permissive act, rather than a compulsory one. This meant that it allowed local authorities to act, but it did not force them to clean up their towns. The Act did not have any authority in London – this was a big weakness.

There was in fact considerable opposition to the 1848 Act. This was because its reforms were expensive to apply. There was also personal opposition to Chadwick himself. He was considered a difficult person to work with. Although he achieved great things, he also made mistakes and upset many important individuals and groups. In 1854, with the worst of the cholera epidemic over, Chadwick's opponents finally got the better of him. When the Public Health Act came up for review in 1854, Chadwick was voted out and was forced to retire. The Board of Health itself was dissolved in 1858.

Despite this failure, matters of public health had made considerable progress in Britain and firm foundations had been laid on which future reformers could build.

TASKS

1. What does Source 16 tell you about the living conditions of the poor in the mid 19th century?
2. Study Source 18. List the threats to health that you can see in the picture.
3. How successful was the Public Health Act of 1848?

Later Victorian health reforms

Cholera returned to Britain again in 1854. However, in that year Dr John Snow made a breakthrough in proving that there was a link between cholera and the water supply. Snow was a London doctor who had developed a particular interest in cholera. He used careful research, observatio n and house-to-house interviews to build up a detailed picture of a limited cholera epidemic that had hit one part of central London – Broad Street, Soho.

SOURCE 19

> The most terrible outbreak of cholera ... took place in Broad Street ... and the adjoining streets, a few weeks ago. Within two hundred and fifty yards ... there were upwards of five hundred fatal attacks ... in ten days. ... The mortality would undoubtedly have been much greater had it not been for the flight of the population.
> ...
> I found that nearly all the deaths had taken place within a short distance of the [water] pump. There were only ten deaths in houses situated decidedly nearer to another street pump. In five of these cases the families ... informed me that they always sent to the pump in Broad Street ... In three other cases, the deceased were children who went to school near the pump in Broad Street. ...
> There is a Brewery in Broad Street, ... and ... I called on Mr Huggins, the proprietor. He informed me that ... none of them [over seventy workmen] had suffered from cholera ... The men are allowed a certain quantity of malt liquor, and Mr Huggins believes they do not drink water at all; and he is quite certain that the workmen never obtained water from the pump in the street. There is a deep well in the brewery

Extracts from Dr John Snow's account On the Mode of Communication of Cholera, *1854, pp. 38-40, 42*

Snow's research discovered that:
- All infected houses got their water from a single pump;
- A local brewery that had not been affected by cholera never used that pump because it had its own water supply;
- A woman living a long way from the area, who had died of cholera, always had water from the Broad Street pump sent to her because she liked the taste.

Snow was given permission to remove the handle of the Broad Street pump and there were no more cases of cholera in the area. When the pump was dug out, it was found that a cesspool just one metre from the pump had seeped its contents into the water supply. Snow published his findings in 1854 and this helped to re-focus the public health debate on water supply.

Central government now realised that it had to work with local authorities to improve public health. They finally accepted one of Chadwick's principal recommendations and appointed Dr John Simon (1816-1904) as Chief Medical Adviser in 1855. He was successful in his role, introducing tough public health regulations.

The smell from London's sewers had long been a problem. During the long, hot summer of 1858 the city suffered what was to become known as the 'Great Stink'.

SOURCE 20

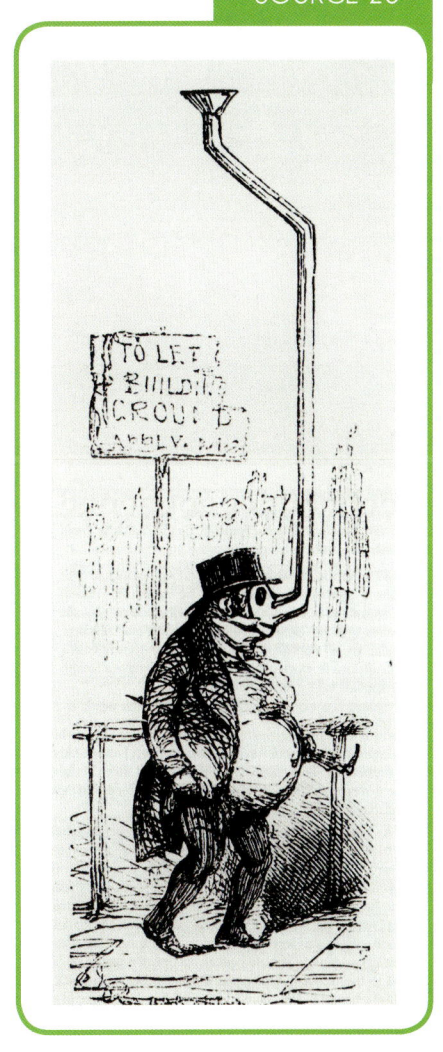

A cartoon of 1849 offering people a way of avoiding the smell of the London sewers by sniffing the purer air further up

One of Chadwick's mistakes had been to order all of London's rubbish and sewage to be flushed into the River Thames, in an attempt to combat cholera. In the summer of 1858 the smell from the filthy River Thames was so bad that Parliament had to be suspended. The Great Stink convinced people that the issue of sanitation had to be dealt with, and steps were taken to improve London's sewerage system.

Joseph Bazalgette (1819-91) proved to be an outstanding pioneer of public health engineering. He oversaw the building of London's new sewerage system from 1859, as well as the Thames Embankment.

SOURCE 21

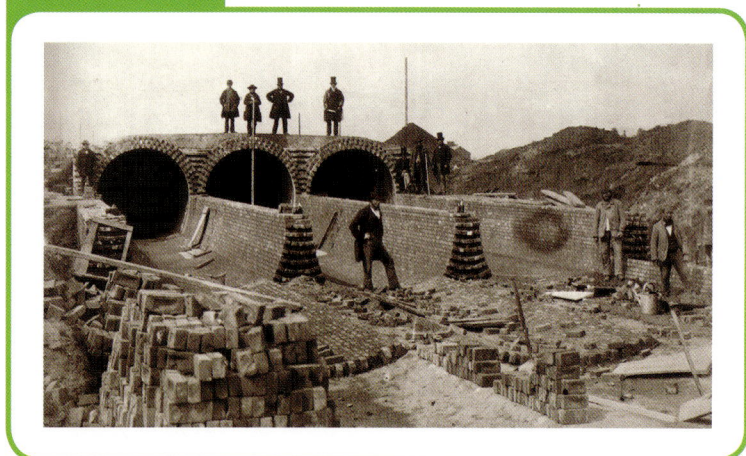

Bazalgette inspecting the building of London's sewers

By 1865 London's sewage, although still dumped in the River Thames, was being deposited downstream, away from the city. The new sewers were very large, as can be seen in Source 21, and could not easily be blocked.

Another cholera epidemic in 1865-66 killed 20,000 people. This allowed Dr John Simon to push through Parliament a Sanitary Act in 1866, which made it compulsory for all local authorities to appoint a Board of Health. However, Dr Simon's most important achievement was the Public Health Act of 1875. This had two key aspects:

- The Act brought together all previous public health measures into one law;
  - The Act was compulsory. By law local authorities now had to provide clean water, proper drainage and sewers, and appoint a Medical Officer of Health.

Chadwick's ideas had at last been accepted and made compulsory. Public health provision had moved away from the *laissez faire* attitude of earlier times to one where central government had become fully involved. Through the efforts of individual people and the health needs of an expanding population, Britain's inhabitants could look forward to a healthier and longer life.

TASKS

1. How important for public health was the work of Dr John Snow and why?
2. What was the 'Great Stink'?
3. Why do you think that the Public Health Act of 1875 was more likely to succeed than the 1848 Act?

DEVELOPMENTS IN PATIENT CARE

Hospitals had traditionally been for the very poor. Wealthy people were treated at home. People who went into hospital often did not come out again or, if they did, their condition was likely to be worse. They caught diseases from other patients or from nurses. Florence Nightingale herself referred to hospitals as 'gateways to death', as standards of nursing were very poor and conditions in hospitals were unhygienic.

We have seen in Chapter 7 that the Christian church had set up hospitals run by monks and nuns in the Middle Ages, and that London had specialist hospitals like St Thomas' and St Bartholomew's, that had been set up voluntarily. Henry VIII closed down the monasteries in Wales and England in the sixteenth century and the monks were forced to leave. From then on, nuns did most of the nursing that was available. This is why certain nurses today are called 'sisters'. However, the quality of nursing care in hospitals was generally poor. Some nurses were simply paupers from the workhouses who were really only cleaners; they had no nursing training and either ignored the patients or treated them badly.

The following sources show how poor the standards were in hospitals.

SOURCE 22

Duo decimo die July ann dm 1712

James Jones Joyner did agree to clear the severall wards within this Hospital of Buggs for five Guineys to be paid him imediately and eight pounds at the years end and if [...] & governors be not at the years end satisfied that he deserves 8 pounds he will leave it to the governors to allow him what they shall think fitt to be accomplished from this day to Micha 1713: memorandum such beds as he takes asunder he is to make good.

St Bartholomew's Hospital, 1712

SOURCE 23

drunkenness was rife among the hospital's staff. Some female nurses, avoiding the hospital's armed guards by using the hospital sewers at low tide, smuggled in rum in pig bladders suspended under their skirts. Staff were accused of stealing patient's food[1]; patients of the '2nd new ward East' petitioned the Admiralty by letter, claiming to be afraid to eat their rations in case they had been poisoned, and to have been threatened with knives by staff of the hospital[2]. A Nurse Brown was dismissed by the Hospital Executive for infecting a number of patients with 'a foul disease', and other nurses were dismissed for not keeping their rooms tidy[3].

[1] (Tait 1906, p 139);
[2] (letter dated 17 December 1761, National Maritime Museum)
[3] (Governing Committee Report Book 1765)

From 'The Royal Hospital Haslar: from Lind to the 21st century', an article by Eric Birbeck, 2011

SOURCE 24

At the Westminster, which I have always considered one of the best though the poorest, I had a head nurse with me last night, (a very admirable woman), and she told me that, in the course of her long life's experience at the Westminster Hospital she had never known a nurse who was not drunken – and that there was immoral conduct practised within the very walls of the ward, of which she gave me some awful instances – so much for our moral Boards.

A letter from Florence Nightingale to her father on 22 February 1854

The most common complaints in the early nineteenth century about nurses who were not nuns was that they were dirty or drunk. Nursing in the mid nineteenth century was not a job that many respectable young ladies would choose.

SOURCE 25

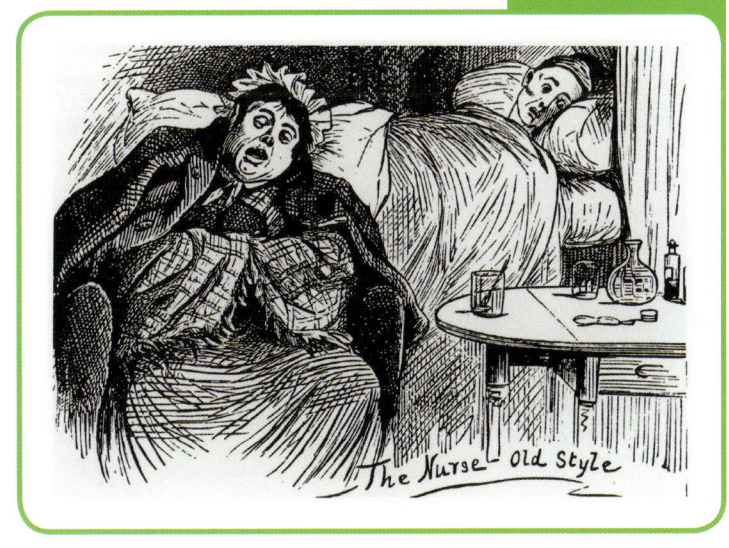

A nineteenth century cartoon showing how a typical nurse was viewed. She is drunk

TASK

1. Use the information in the sources above to describe the standard of nursing in the eighteenth and early nineteenth centuries.

The work of Florence Nightingale

Florence Nightingale (1820-1910) was a respectable lady from a wealthy family, who did more than anyone else at the time to improve the standards of hospitals and nursing. Despite the opposition of her family, she trained as a nurse in Germany and in Paris in 1851-52. By 1854 she was working in the Middlesex Hospital during yet another cholera epidemic.

In 1854 the British government was being heavily criticised for the conduct of the Crimean War. *The Times* newspaper reported regularly on the military mismanagement, but also revealed the disgusting state of the British military hospital. Nightingale wrote to Sidney Herbert, Minister of War Supplies, who was an old family friend, volunteering to help in the Crimea. By coincidence, her letter crossed in the post with a letter from Sidney Herbert, asking her to do just that. With government money and 38 of the best nurses she could find, Florence Nightingale set out for the British military hospital at Scutari on the Black Sea coast of Turkey.

When Florence arrived at the hospital, she found the conditions horrendous. There were 1,700 patients: some were casualties of battle but the vast majority were victims of typhoid and cholera. There was filth and vermin everywhere. There were not enough beds or medical supplies and patients were dying in their scores.

SOURCE 26

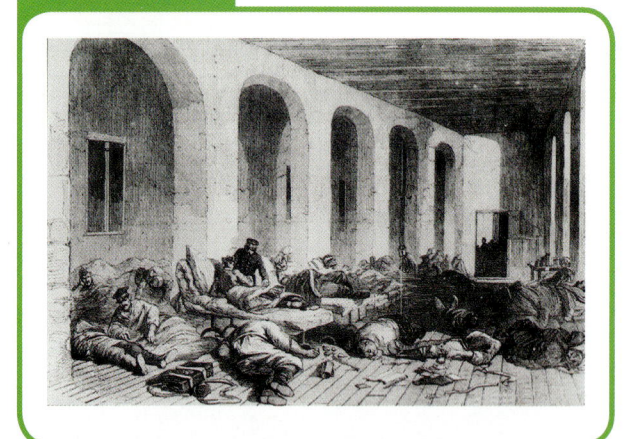

Conditions in the military hospital at Scutari in 1854 before the arrival of Florence Nightingale

The army doctors opposed Florence Nightingale and resented her interference. However, she had plenty of support – from Sidney Herbert and from Dr Andrew Smith, head of the Army Medical Department. Dr Smith made sure that she received sufficient supplies of the items that she needed. She also had money and the backing of *The Times*, which drummed up public support for this determined, energetic woman.

Nightingale obtained soap and water and made sure that the patients were washed. She set up a laundry and obtained new clothing for them. She persuaded the Army Supply Corps to provide food and medicines. She also made sure that the wards were cleaned and she separated patients who were suffering from different complaints in order to prevent the spread of disease.

The results of Florence Nightingale's work were extraordinary. After just six months, only 100 patients were still confined to bed in Scutari Hospital. The death rate at the hospital was reduced from 42% to 2%. The wards had been transformed and so had Florence Nightingale's reputation. This was a turning point in the development of nursing care.

SOURCE 27

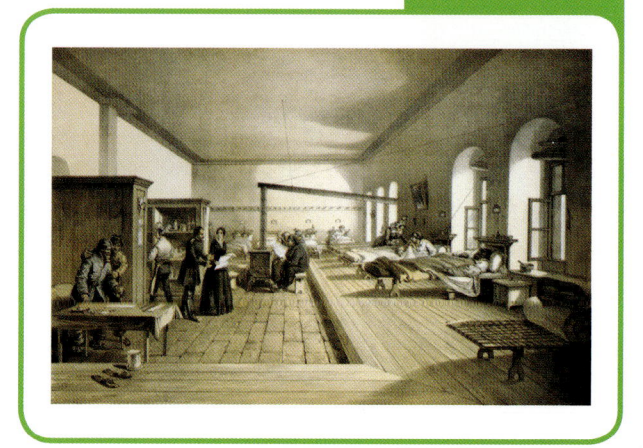

A hospital ward at Scutari after Florence Nightingale had made her improvements

A report in *The Times* newspaper described Nightingale as a 'ministering angel', who was a welcome sight to the sick and injured soldiers in the hospital. It told of how, every night after the doctors and other staff had left, she would visit all the patients as she made her rounds by the light of a small lamp. As a result of this report she became affectionately known as 'the Lady with the Lamp'.

Florence Nightingale was not the only nurse who worked hard to improve conditions for injured soldiers during the Crimean War of 1854-56. Betsi Cadwaladr and Mary Seacole also travelled to the battlefields in order to care for British soldiers. Their contributions to nursing and patient care during the conflict are also very important.

Betsi Cadwaladr

SOURCE 28

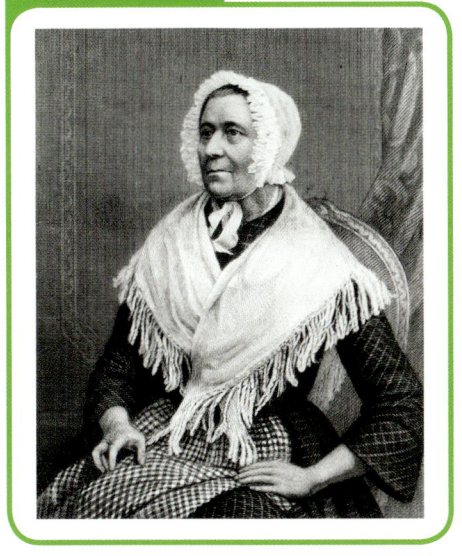

An engraving of Betsi Cadwaladr

Betsi Cadwaladr (1789-1860) was born in Bala, north Wales, one of 16 children. She became a servant in Liverpool at the age of 14 and here she learned to read, write and to speak English. She now called herself Elizabeth Davies, a name that would be easier for English-speaking people to pronounce. Her work as a maid for a sea captain allowed her to travel the world. She also took care of the sick and delivered babies whilst on board ship.

Betsi qualified as a nurse late in life after training in a London hospital. In 1854 at the age of 65 she made her way to the Crimea to help nurse the wounded soldiers there, but Florence Nightingale kept her waiting at Scutari for many frustrating weeks. Betsi then made her own way to the port of Balaclava on the Black Sea. Here she showed that she would do anything to improve the quality of care for her patients.

Betsi strongly disliked the bureaucracy that Florence Nightingale had set up; she felt that this served to deprive the wounded soldiers of food, clothing and even bandages. She cleaned wounds and changed dressings, working every day from 6 a.m. to 11 p.m. She fought against the system and when Florence Nightingale witnessed what she had achieved at Balaclava, she was won over to her ways. Betsi left the Crimea in 1855, aged 66, suffering from cholera and dysentery.

The Betsi Cadwaladr NHS Trust in north Wales was named after this remarkable woman.

Mary Seacole

Mary Seacole (1805-81) was born in Kingston, Jamaica. Her mother was a free black woman and her father was a Scottish soldier. Her mother owned a hotel in Kingston, which was also used as a medical centre by British soldiers and sailors. Here Mary helped her mother to nurse British soldiers and she watched the army surgeons carefully. As a result she became a good herbalist and a competent surgeon.

Mary travelled to London in 1854. Like Florence Nightingale and Betsi Cadwaladr, she wanted to help in the Crimean War. She felt that her experience in tropical medicine would be invaluable. Using her own money, Mary travelled to the Crimea, visiting Florence Nightingale on the way. In 1855 she opened the 'British Hotel' between Balaclava and Sebastopol. Here soldiers were able to buy food and medicine and Mary would deal with their medical complaints. She even went onto the battlefield to help the wounded.

When the Crimean War ended in 1856 most of Mary Seacole's food and stock had to be left behind. Soon after returning to London she was declared bankrupt. In 1857 she published her autobiography, which played its part in raising public awareness of the contribution of nursing during the conflict.

SOURCE 29

Head-Quarters, Camp, Crimea, June 30, 1856
I have much pleasure in bearing testimony to Mrs Seacole's kindness and attention to the sick of the Railway Labourers' Army Works Corps and Land Transport Corps during the winters of 1854 and 1855.
She not only, from the knowledge she had acquired in the West Indies, was enabled to administer appropriate remedies for their ailments, but, what was of as much or more importance, she charitably furnished them with proper nourishment, which they had no means of obtaining except in the hospital, and most of that class had an objection to go into hopsital, particularly the railway labourers and the men of the Army Works Corps

JOHN HALL,
Inspector-General of Hospitals

From Wonderful Adventures of Mrs Seacole in Many Lands, *Mary Seacole, Penguin Classics, 2005, p. 114*

TASKS

1. Explain why Florence Nightingale is known as 'The Lady with the Lamp'.
2. Use Sources 26 and 27 to show how hospital conditions changed during the Crimean War.
3. How successful was Florence Nightingale?
4. Describe the work of Betsi Cadwaladr as a nurse.
5. Describe the contribution of Mary Seacole to nursing.

Hospitals and the development of nursing

Florence Nightingale was greeted as a national heroine when she returned to England at the end of the Crimean War. She spent the next four years (1856-60) campaigning to reform army medical services. She wrote an 800-page report to the government, listing what needed to be changed in order to improve patient care. The list included fresh air, clean floors, better food, trained nurses and plenty of light in purpose-built hospitals.

In 1859 Florence Nightingale published her best-selling *Notes on Nursing*, which sold 15,000 copies in the first month and went through many editions. *The Times* newspaper set up a Nightingale Fund, which raised £50,000. In 1860 she used this money to set up training schools for nurses at St Thomas' Hospital and at King's College Hospital in London. Here nurses were trained to run hospitals according to Florence Nightingale's principles. They were trained to be as clean as possible, to change dressings and to be proper assistants to doctors and surgeons.

Nightingale Nurses were a separate and important new branch of the medical profession. Instead of simply being minders or cleaners, as in the past, they were now a central part of the patient's care and treatment. Florence Nightingale's principles were first taken up in the voluntary hospitals, but by the mid 1860s they were spreading more widely. Whenever new hospitals were built, designers would ask for her advice, as when the Royal Liverpool Infirmary was built between 1887 and 1889.

At the end of the nineteenth century, many other cities and towns built their own new hospitals. Smaller towns built their own 'cottage hospitals'. In some cases, hospitals specialising in particular branches of care began to appear. Hospitals for infectious diseases were built, usually in isolated locations. Other hospitals specialised in infections of the ear, nose and throat. Specialist eye hospitals were also created at this time.

Without doubt, the basic standard of hospital care had risen enormously by the end of the nineteenth century. The wealthier classes, who could afford to choose, were now more prepared to go into hospital for treatment, rather than be treated at home. In addition, nursing was now seen as a respectable career, with real prospects.

In 1830 there had been no trained nurses in Britain; in 1900 there were 68,000. In 1899 the International Council of Nurses was founded in London. Nursing was becoming recognised as a profession, largely due to the efforts of Florence Nightingale.

TASKS

1. Draw a spider diagram to show Florence Nightingale's contribution to nursing after her return from the Crimean War.
2. Describe how far nursing had changed by 1900.

Examination practice

This section provides further guidance on how to answer Question 1(b), 2(b) and 3(b) from Unit 3. It asks for a discription and is worth 4 marks.

Question 1(b), 2(b), 3(b) – the understanding of a key feature through the selection of appropriate knowledge

Describe the achievement of Florence Nightingale in the nineteenth century.

[4 marks]

Tips on how to answer

- Make sure that you only include information that is **directly relevant**.
- Jot down your initial thoughts, **making a brief list** of the points you intend to mention.
- After you have finished your list, try to put the points into **chronological order** by numbering them.
- It is a good idea to start your answer **using words from the question**, e.g. 'Florence Nightingale's achievement in the nineteenth century…'
- Try to include **specific factual details** such as dates, events, the names of key people and important ideas. The more informed your description, the higher the mark you will receive.
- Aim to write a **good-sized paragraph**.

Response by candidate one

Florence Nightingale worked as a nurse in the Crimean War and improved the standard of nursing there. She set up training schools for nurses in England and improved hospitals.

Examiner's comment

This is a very generalised answer with weak points made. There is a lack of factual detail. This is a Level One answer, which would score only half marks (2 marks).

Response by candidate two

800-page report (4), parental opposition (1), Crimean War (2), training schools (6), consulted on design (7), Lady with the Lamp (3), 'Notes on Nursing' (6)

Florence Nightingale was a respectable lady from a wealthy family and she trained as a nurse despite the opposition of her parents. Nursing was looked down upon at that time. In 1854 Florence volunteered to go to help in the Crimean War. Here she found the military hospital at Scutari in a dreadful condition. She improved standards considerably so that the death rate was reduced from 42% to 2%. This was an incredible achievement. Florence's caring attitude, keeping an eye on her patients at night, earned her the affectionate title of 'The Lady with the Lamp'.

On her return to England Florence wrote an 800-page report to the government, listing the changes that were needed to improve patient care. She also published her 'Notes on Nursing', which was a best seller. 'The Times' newspaper set up the Nightingale Fund and this collected £50,000. Florence was able to use this money to set up training schools for nurses. Whenever new hospitals were built, designers would ask Florence for her advice. Her achievement was to improve nursing considerably by the end of the nineteenth century, turning it into an acceptable profession.

Examiner's comment

This is a very detailed and accurate description of the achievement of Florence Nightingale in the nineteenth century. The candidate has given prior thought to the details needed for the answer and has clearly identified the relevant factors, which have been placed in correct chronological order. These have been presented in a way that shows clear understanding. This is a full Level Two answer, worth maximum (4) marks.

Now you have a go

Describe Edwin Chadwick's achievement in the nineteenth century.

[4 marks]

CHAPTER 9

HOW HAS HEALTH CARE IN WALES AND ENGLAND IMPROVED FROM THE TWENTIETH CENTURY TO TODAY?

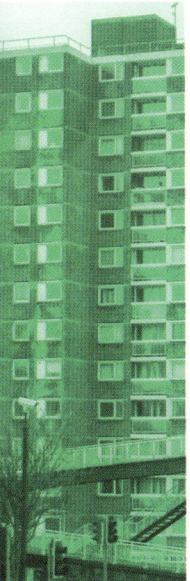

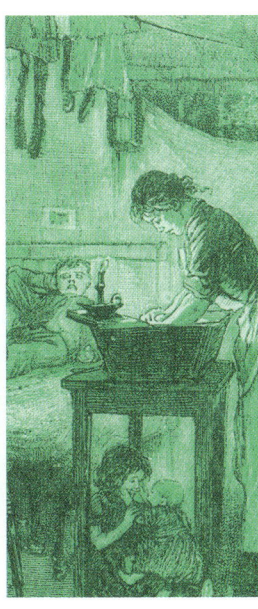

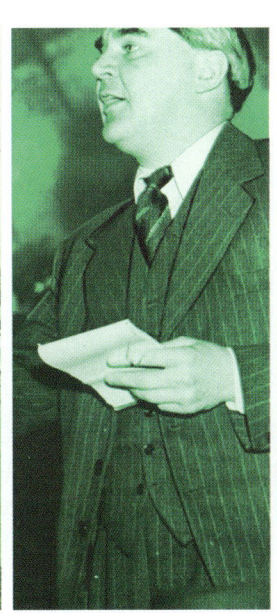

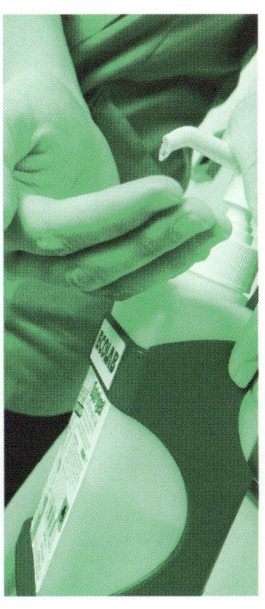

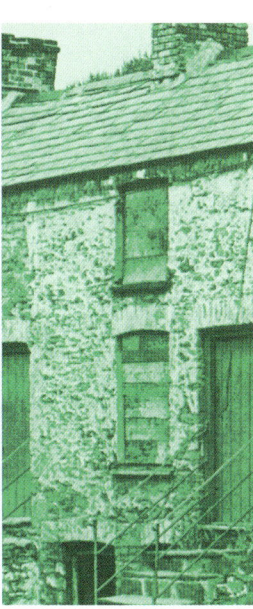

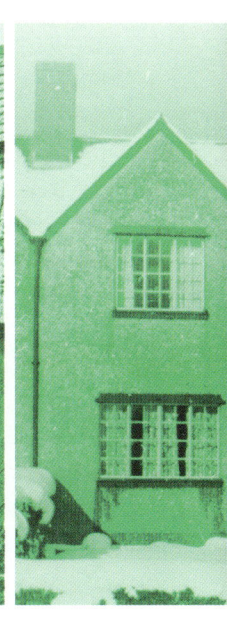

ATTEMPTS TO PROVIDE HEALTHIER HOUSING AND CLEANER AIR

Housing for working people in the nineteenth century had generally been very poor. The atmosphere and the environment in industrial towns and cities had often been heavily polluted. Life for working people had been unhealthy on the whole.

The banning of back-to-back housing

Back-to-back housing had been very popular in fast-growing industrial towns because it allowed more houses to be packed into valuable sites. The houses were very unhealthy, as the buildings lacked through ventilation. This was highlighted during the recurring cholera epidemics of the nineteenth century.

One option for improving back-to-back housing was to 'cut through' each pair of houses, making one good house. This has been done to good effect in Llanidloes, a former woollen industrial town in mid Wales.

A more radical alternative was to ban the further building of back-to-back houses and then to knock down existing ones. This resulted in many of these houses being demolished in industrial towns in England in the 1920s. However at Newtown, another former woollen industrial town in mid Wales, such housing still existed until the 1960s.

SOURCE 1

Victoria Avenue, Llanidloes – a row of former back-to-back houses

103

'Homes for heroes'

At the start of the twentieth century house building was lagging behind population growth. The First World War slowed down the process even further. By 1918 there was a serious housing shortage in Britain. Many houses were unfit for people to live in.

At the end of the First World War, Prime Minister David Lloyd George declared that the slums would be swept away and replaced with 'homes fit for heroes'. This promise proved to be very optimistic.

The Housing Act of 1919 offered government grants to local councils to help them provide homes for families with low incomes. Private builders could also qualify for financial assistance if they built houses that could be let at low rents. This compares with the need to provide 'affordable housing' today. At the same time, local authorities were told to carry out surveys of their housing needs and act to remedy shortages.

From 1919 until the 1930s, when the Great Depression occurred, estates of council houses sprang up all over Britain. These estates were often plain and monotonous to look at, but all the houses had gardens, inside lavatories and bathrooms, and were far superior to most previous working-class houses.

SOURCE 2

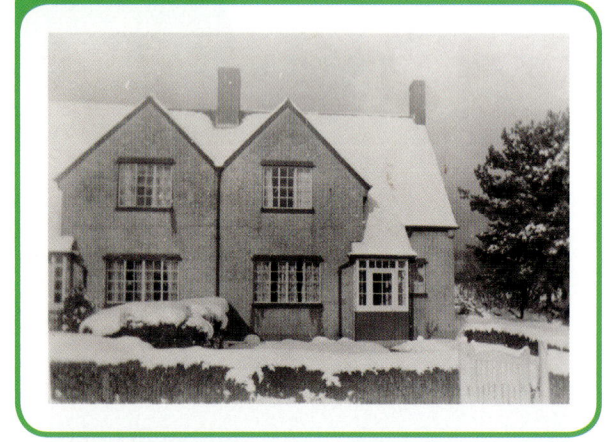

Council houses built near Cardigan, west Wales, in 1923

Slum clearance

In 1930 a special grant was offered to local authorities to carry out slum clearance. The aim was not just to pull down slum housing but to re-house their inhabitants as well. So the grant payment was only made if the occupants of the demolished houses were provided with alternative accommodation at rents they 'could reasonably be expected to pay'. In 1933 councils were asked to prepare five-year programmes for the abolition of slums. Although there was great activity in some places, the Second World War put a stop to progress. In 1939 there were still half a million dwellings classed as slums in Wales and England.

In 1942 the Beveridge Report was published. This provided a Plan for Reconstruction after the Second World War. The report highlighted 'Five Evil Giants' that would have to be addressed after the war was over: Want, Idleness, Disease, Ignorance and Squalor. Beveridge stated that squalor could be addressed with 'more and better houses'.

During the Second World War (1939-1945) German bombing destroyed half a million homes in Britain. This resulted in a desperate housing shortage, which was even more serious than that of 1918. Aneurin Bevan was the Minister for Health and Housing in the post-war Labour government. He severely restricted private building and directed building efforts towards providing more council houses. Grants were given to local councils so that they could build at lower than normal cost and charge lower rents. One and a quarter million new homes were built by 1951, but much still needed to be done. One third of all homes in Wales and England in 1951 had no fixed bath; more than one million houses had no flush toilet.

As the needs of the housing shortage were addressed throughout the 1950s, slum clearance continued. An act of parliament in 1956 discontinued all government grants to local authorities, except those for slum clearance. In the 1960s, many inner-city slums were cleared and replaced by high-rise blocks of flats.

SOURCE 3

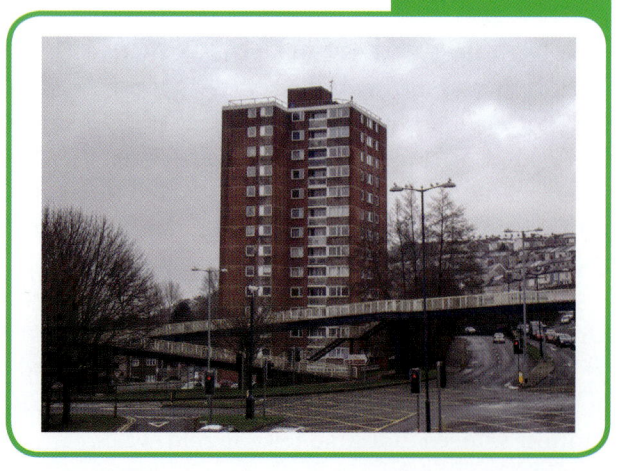

A tower block in Dyfatty Street, Swansea, built in the 1960s

The Clean Air Act, 1956

The post-war Labour governments had realised the need for improved health and the associated importance of clean air. In 1949 they passed the Access to the Countryside Act to encourage the general public to enjoy life outside the towns and cities, and to enjoy the clean air of the countryside.

SOURCE 4

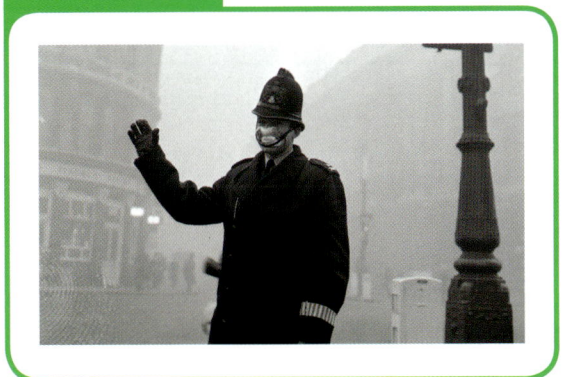

A policeman in London during the Great Smog, December 1952

The air in many industrial towns and cities continued to be polluted, well into the twentieth century. Cities like Birmingham and Sheffield, for example, continuously had a haze of pollution hanging over them. London was notorious for its **smog**, which was a heavy fog containing smoke and gases. In December 1952 the Great Smog fell over London. At least 4,000 people died of respiratory illness brought on by the smog, making it the worst health disaster in London since the influenza epidemic of 1918. The smog was so thick that it stopped trains, cars and public events.

The Great Smog speeded up action to reduce air pollution. In 1956 the Clean Air Act was passed and remained in force until 1964. The Act introduced smokeless zones in cities where only smokeless fuels could be burned. The use of cleaner coals, electricity and gas was encouraged for heating. This reduced the amount of smoke pollution and sulphur dioxide that had previously been emitted from dirty coal fires in houses. The Act also included measures to relocate power stations away from cities.

The Clean Air Act of 1956 was also an important milestone in protecting Britain's environment. The Great Smog of 1952 may well have inspired the modern environmental movement in Britain. The 1956 Act led to the 1968 Clean Air Act so that, by 1971, the amount of smoke pollution entering the atmosphere in Britain had been reduced by 65%.

TASKS

1. Use Source 1 to describe how back-to-back housing was improved.
2. Describe what was meant by 'homes for heroes'.
3. How important was the Clean Air Act of 1956?

THE ESTABLISHMENT OF THE NATIONAL HEALTH SERVICE

The Beveridge Report of 1942 had highlighted Five Evil Giants that needed to be addressed for reconstruction after the Second World War was over. We have seen that one of the Giants was Squalor; another was Disease. Beveridge suggested that disease could be addressed through a 'free National Health Service'. This suggestion was very appealing to very many people and 600,000 copies of the Beveridge Report were sold.

By 1944 the new National Health system was being planned. It was to be available to all and was to cover all necessary forms of health care. In 1945 a new Labour government was elected. It was determined to apply the ideas of the Beveridge Report, especially with regard to health.

SOURCE 5

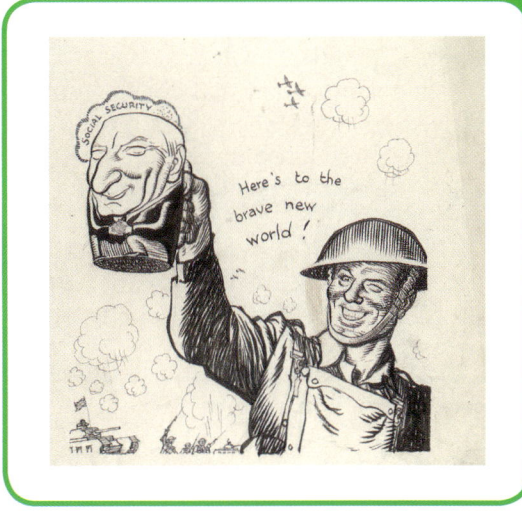

A cartoon in the Daily Mirror *newspaper welcoming the Beveridge Report, 2 December 1942*

SOURCE 6

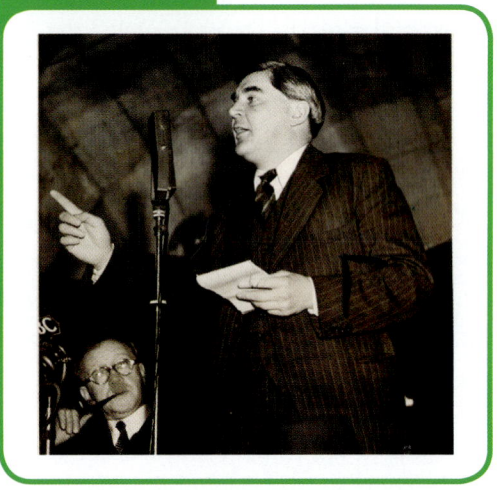

Aneurin Bevan, Minister for Health 1945-51

Aneurin Bevan, Labour MP for Ebbw Vale in south Wales, was appointed Minister for Health. His main task was to oversee the establishment of the National Health Service that would care for British citizens 'from cradle to grave'. Bevan had been born in Tredegar where the Tredegar Workingmen's Medical Aid Society had been established to provide free medical aid and hospital treatment in return for a small weekly subscription. The Society had operated like a miniature National Health Service. As Minister for Health, Bevan's first challenge was to get the support of the public for setting up a National Health Service.

SOURCE 7

medical treatment ... should be made available to rich and poor alike in accordance with medical need and by no other criteria. ... financial anxiety in time of sickness is a serious hindrance to recovery, apart from its unnecessary cruelty. ... no society can legitimately call itself civilized if a sick person is denied medical aid because of lack of means. ...
   The records show that it is the mother in the average family who suffers most from the absence of a free health service. In trying to balance her domestic budget she puts her own needs last. ...
   The essence of a satisfactory health service is that the rich and the poor are treated alike, that poverty is not a disability, and wealth is not advantaged.

From In Place of Fear *by Aneurin Bevan, 1990*

Aneurin Bevan was successful in getting support for his proposals and in 1946 the National Health Service Act was passed.

The National Health Service Act, 1946

SOURCE 8

The National Health Service Act of 1946 is perhaps the best known of all Labour's post-war social reforms. Its aim was to set up a health service that shall be 'free of charge' and available to everyone. This was a radical change.

Historian Roger Turvey, writing in Wales and Britain, 1906-51, *1997*

The NHS Act certainly had its supporters but it also had its critics.
- Under the NHS 3,000 hospitals would be nationalised. This was opposed by local authorities and by voluntary bodies that ran the hospitals;
- The NHS was going to be hugely expensive to run;
- The strongest opposition came from the British Medical Association (BMA), which represented the medical profession. Doctors didn't want to become government employees and they didn't want to see their income reduced.

SOURCE 9

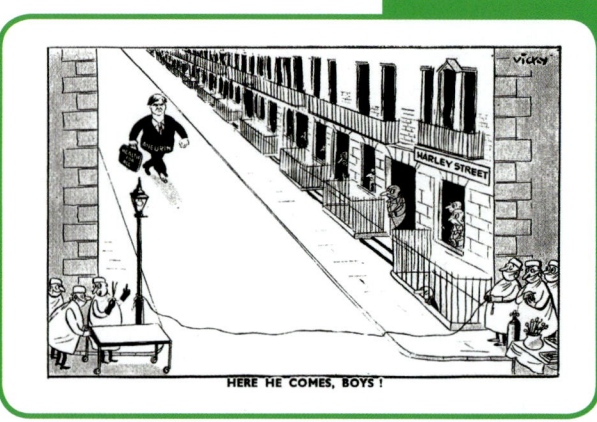

A cartoon published in the Daily Mirror *newspaper, 7 August 1945, showing the opposition of doctors*

Aneurin Bevan had a powerful personality and was very persuasive. He eventually managed to win the majority of the medical profession over to his ideas. He gained the support of hospital consultants by promising them a salary and by allowing them to treat private patients in NHS hospitals. Opposition to his proposals crumbled and when the NHS was finally introduced in July 1948, more than 90% of doctors had enrolled in the service.

The government had to explain to the people what the NHS offered them and newspapers reacted positively to the new service.

Terms of the NHS Act:
- Hospitals were nationalised under the Ministry of Health and were organized into regional groups or health authorities;
- Consultants in hospitals received salaries and all treatment to patients in hospitals was free;
- A national system of GPs was provided and they, along with dentists and opticians, received fees according to the numbers of patients on their registers, not according to the treatment given. Again, treatment was free to the patient;
- Local authorities were paid to provide vaccinations, maternity care, district nurses, health visitors and ambulances. Local Authority health centres were introduced for the first time.

SOURCE 10

On Monday morning you will wake up in a new Britain – in a State which "takes over" all citizens six months before they are born, provides cash and free services for their birth, for their early years, their schooling, sickness, workless days, widowhood, and retirement. Finally, it helps defray the cost of their departure. All this, with free doctoring, dentistry, and medicine ... for 4s. 11d. [25p] out of your weekly wage packet

Extract from the Daily Mail *newspaper, 3 July 1948*

TASKS

1. How important was the Beveridge Report for the NHS?
2. Describe the role of Aneurin Bevan in setting up the NHS.
3. Use the information in Source 9 to explain why doctors opposed the NHS.
4. Use Source 10 to explain why the introduction of the NHS was popular.

Benefits for individuals and for society

The demand for health care under the new NHS exceeded all predictions. As soon as the NHS started, the number of patients on doctors' registers rose to 30 million. Patients immediately took advantage of what the NHS had to offer.

The NHS had budgeted £2 million for free spectacles in the first nine months, but this had been spent within six weeks. In 1947, doctors gave out 7 million prescriptions every month; by 1951 the figure had risen to 19 million. By 1949, 8.5 million people had received free dental treatment.

For the first time, poorer people gained access to doctors and to a range of treatments that they previously could not afford. They also had the huge psychological boost of not having to worry about illness or injury. However it was not only the poor who benefitted. Aneurin Bevan had said that he wanted the NHS to treat everyone, and the middle-classes made full use of the service too.

From the 1950s onwards, the extent and quality of the treatment offered by the NHS got better and better. The number of doctors doubled by 1973 and the role of the family doctors was transformed as they increasingly worked as part of teams offering a whole range of health services. Since the establishment of the NHS, hospitals have carried out longer and more complex operations. Some types of transplant surgery have become commonplace; fertility treatment for childless couples has been introduced; vaccination programmes have protected children from illnesses that can kill, like whooping cough, measles, TB and diphtheria.

SOURCE 11

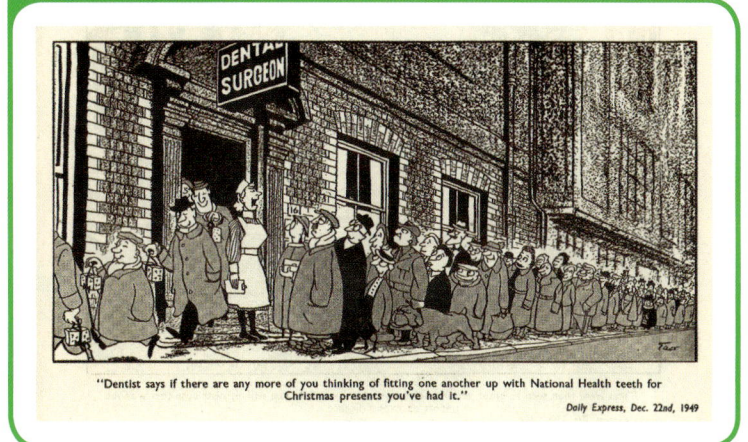

A cartoon showing the enormous take-up of free NHS dental treatment, 1948

The NHS has had a huge impact on the nation's health. Women in particular have benefitted. Before 1948 women had limited access to health care. From the beginning, the NHS made women's health a priority and has continued to do so. Women are now four times more likely to consult a doctor than men and life expectancy has risen from 66 to 82 since 1948.

Services provided by the NHS

- *Emergency and urgent care* – this is provided by Accident and Emergency departments at larger hospitals, by ambulance services and by Minor Injury Units (MIUs) in most hospitals;
- *Hospital services* – these are run and managed by NHS Trusts that make sure that hospitals provide quality health care. Apart from emergency care, hospital care is arranged through a GP, a dentist or an optician. Treatment is free;
- *Dental services* – gums, and a mouth free from disease, are important. To achieve this, the NHS tries to enable everyone to access good quality dental services at a reasonable cost. However there is a shortage of NHS dentists in some areas;
- *GP services* – GPs provide a wide range of family health services: advice on health problems; vaccinations; examinations and treatment; prescriptions for medicines; referrals to other health services and to social services;
- *Eye care services* – NHS 'opticians' include optometrists and dispensing opticians. Optometrists carry out sight tests to check the quality of vision and eye health; dispensing opticians fit glasses and contact lenses;
- *Pharmacies* – as well as providing medicines, pharmacies can offer advice on common problems such as coughs, colds, aches and pains, as well as on healthy eating and on giving up smoking. They can also help to decide whether a person needs to see a doctor. Prescriptions are free in Wales, but in England pharmacies charge £7.65 for each one (2013);
- *Social care services* – these look after the health and welfare of the population. The main groups using this service include children or families who are under stress, people with disabilities or psychological difficulties, people with financial or housing problems and older people who need help with daily living activities;
- *Mental health services* – mental illnesses accounts for one third of all illness in Wales and England. While some are much more severe than others, the impact of these illnesses is often underestimated. If left untreated they can lead to unemployment, the break-up of families, homelessness and even suicide. The NHS believes it is very important that mental health problems are treated.

TASKS

1. Study Source 11. What does it tell you about about the popularity of the early NHS?
2. How has the NHS developed since the 1950s?
3. Draw a spider diagram to show the different services provided by the NHS.

TODAY'S CONCERNS REGARDING HEALTH CARE

With an ever-broadening programme of treatments and an expanding and ageing population, health care in Britain is becoming more and more expensive. Against this background, the NHS has to justify its costs and face up to radical reforms in order to be affordable.

Costs of health care

The initial critics of the high cost of the NHS when it was set up in 1948 were soon proved to be correct. In order to meet the immediate unexpectedly high costs, prescription charges were introduced in 1951. Charges for other services such as dental treatment for those aged over 21 and contributions towards the cost of spectacles were also introduced. Aneurin Bevan, who is regarded as the 'architect' of the NHS, resigned from the government as a protest against these charges. He said that they were against the principles of a free health service.

Following devolution in 1999, the Welsh Government became responsible for the NHS in Wales and since then it has been the responsibility of the Welsh Minister for Health and Social Services. By the start of the twenty first century the costs of running the

NHS were enormous. For NHS Wales the budget for 2005-6 was £4.9 billion. This was nearly double the amount adopted by the Welsh Assembly when it came into existence in 1999. Almost 40% of the total Welsh Government budget is spent on health care and about 75,000 people (6.5% of the Welsh workforce) are employed by NHS Wales. In 2008-9 the cost of running the NHS in England was £48 billion. This was an increase of £4 billion on 2007-8.

Although the running costs are very high, research has shown that the cost of treating people on the NHS is lower than in countries that operate other systems of health care.

SOURCE 12

the fact remains that the NHS costs less than other systems. For example, the USA has a private health care system which costs 12 per cent of national income while the NHS costs just 6 per cent.

Historians I. Dawson and I. Coulson, writing in Medicine and Health through Time, *2000*

Greater life expectancy

Life expectancy in the UK has reached its highest level on record for both men and women. A newborn baby boy in 2010 could expect to live for 78.1 years and a newborn baby girl 82.1 years.

SOURCE 13

	At birth		At age 65	
	Males	Females	Males	Females
United Kingdom	78.1	82.1	17.8	20.4
England	78.4	82.4	18.0	20.6
Wales	77.5	81.7	17.5	20.1
Scotland	75.8	80.3	16.6	19.2
Northern Ireland	77.0	81.4	17.3	20.1

Source: Office for National Statistics: Interim Life Tables 2008-2010
Figures have been rounded to one decimal place.

Life expectancy at birth and at age 65, UK and constituent countries, 2008-2010

The table above shows that, within the UK, life expectancy varies by country. England has the highest life expectancy at birth: 78.4 for males and 82.4 for females. The comparable figures for Wales are: 77.5 and 81.7.

Females continue to live longer than males, but the gap has been closing, having narrowed from 6.0 years to 4.0 years since 1948. Life expectancy is expected to increase even further, both for males and for females. This will be an added concern and challenge for the provision of health care in Britain.

On-going NHS reforms

In 2003, 22 Local Health Boards (LHBs) were set up in Wales, corresponding to the 22 local authorities. The boards would develop and provide the appropriate health service for the local area. In October 2009, they were reorganized into seven LHBs, which together cover the whole of Wales. In 2005, the then Welsh Assembly Government published a strategy for health and social care in Wales by 2015, called 'Designed for Life'. This aims to change the NHS "from the national illness service it currently is into a truly national health service".

In July 2010 Britain's coalition government published its proposals for NHS health reforms in England. They called their proposals 'Equity and Excellence: Liberating the NHS'. This was followed by the Health and Social Care Bill. The government's idea was to devolve much of the NHS budget to groups of doctors and to introduce more competition into health care. The Health and Social Care Bill caused much debate and the government had to make several alterations to it. The proposals are intended to shake up the NHS and to radically restructure it.

The Guardian newspaper summarised the reasons why the government planned to shake up the NHS in England:

SOURCE 14

The health secretary ... says that while the NHS is world-class in some respects, and employs leading medical figures, it is still not good enough in some key areas of care. "For example ... rates of mortality for some respiratory diseases and some cancers, and some measures of stroke, have been among the worst in the developed world. International evidence also shows the NHS has much further to go on managing care more effectively," says the Department of Health. Doctors have cast doubt on the evidence ... about the quality of NHS care, and critics argue that [the health secretary's] "modernisation" changes will usher in widespread privatisation of NHS services.

'NHS reforms: what will happen and why',
The Guardian, *16 March 2011*

The Guardian claimed that the government's proposals would arguably bring about the most radical restructuring of the NHS since its creation in 1948. The newspaper later reported that England's 150 or so Primary Care Trusts (PCTs) will be wound up in 2013 and their work will pass to groups of GPs, called General Practice Commissioning Consortiums (GPCCs), each with its own budget. The consortiums will agree contracts with hospitals and other health providers and will have a total of £80 billion of NHS funds.

The government believes that GPs know their patients and their local hospitals and so are best placed to decide on treatments. Getting rid of 24,000 PCT jobs will save money. The proposals were still being discussed in 2012 because they are such radical measures.

Hospital Acquired Infections

There has been much criticism in recent years of hospital cleanliness. An associated concern for health care has been the problem of dealing with Hospital Acquired Infections (HAIs). These are infections that were not present when a patient went in to hospital. Patients are now tested for infections before being admitted. There are two major infections that are causing concern:
- MRSA (Methicillin-resistant Staphylococcus aureus) – this is a bacterium responsible for several infections in humans that are difficult to treat. It is especially troublesome for patients who have open wounds, invasive devices inserted into them, or have weakened immune systems. Some strains of MRSA are resistant to antibiotics, but an effective drug now used is Vancomycin;
- C-Diff (Clostridium Difficile) – this is a bacterium that causes severe diarrhoea and other intestinal illnesses. The bacterium is present in the gut of a small percentage of the adult population and other people may accidentally absorb the spores of the bacterium while they are patients in hospital. If the bacterium enters the colon, it can spread and cause intense abdominal pain, which might even be fatal. Antibiotics like Vancomycin are effective against C-Diff.

In 2004 the NHS introduced its 'Clean Your Hands' campaign where, in addition to advice on thorough hand washing, alcohol-based hand rubs are placed throughout hospitals for use by staff, patients and visitors. This campaign has helped to reduce the number of HAIs significantly.

SOURCE 15

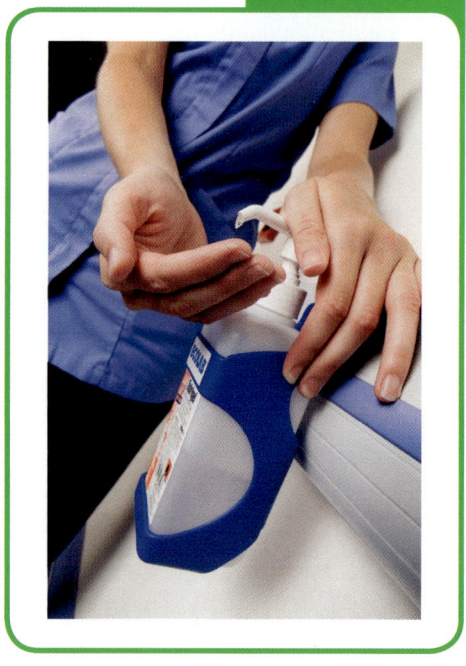

The NHS 'Clean Your Hands' campaign

Care in the Community

This is a policy of treating and caring for physically and mentally disabled people in their homes, rather than in an institution. It has been called 'de-institutionalisation'. Care in institutions was severely criticised during the 1960s and 1970s. In the 1980s a report called 'Making a Reality of Community Care' was published, which outlined the advantages of care in the community and convinced the government of the time to adopt a new policy. In 1988 the government published their own report, 'Community Care: Agenda for Action' and this led to the Community Care Act of 1990. This Act came into force in 1993.

SOURCE 16

Care in the community represented the biggest political change in mental healthcare in the history of the NHS.

It was the result both of social changes and political expediency and a movement away from the isolation of the mentally ill in old Victorian asylums towards their integration into the community.

The aim was to "normalise" the mentally ill and to remove the stigma of a condition that is said to afflict one in four of the British population at some time in their lives.

Extract from a BBC Report, 'The origins of community care', 13 October 1999

The main aim of community care has always been to keep individuals in their own homes wherever possible, rather than provide care in a long-stay institution or residential home. It had come to be accepted that this policy was the best option from a humanitarian and moral perspective. It was also cheaper than the previous system.

However, the care in the community reforms have met with a mixed response. In some cases, community care has failed to provide proper support for people confined to their homes, due to a lack of funding and care workers. This has often led to them feeling isolated and lonely. In a very small minority of cases people with mental health problems, who had previously been in psychiatric hospitals, have committed acts of violence against members of the public, including murder. Such patients should have been assigned a specific care worker, but some had 'slipped through the net', possibly due to a lack of trained staff. This cast doubt on the Care in the Community policy that has undoubtedly benefitted many former residents of out-of-date institutions.

TASKS

1. Use the information in this section to explain why the government thinks that reform of the NHS is necessary.
2. Describe the policy of 'Care in the Community' in your own words.
3. How successful do you think the NHS has been in dealing with today's concerns regarding health care?

Essay question
Have standards in public health and patient care always improved from the Middle Ages to the present day?

[10 marks]

You may wish to discuss the following in your answer:
- *The effectiveness of methods of combating the Black Death;*
- *The impact of industrialisation;*
- *The contributions of Edwin Chadwick and Florence Nightingale;*
- *The establishment and benefits of the NHS;*

and any other relevant factors.
(For advice on answering this question, see page 73.)

Timeline

1. Construct a timeline showing some of the major changes in public health and patient care from the late Middle Ages to the present day.
2. Which change do you think was the most important? Explain your answer fully.

Examination practice

Here is an opportunity for you to practise some of the questions that have been explained in previous chapters.

SECTION A

These examples are taken from Section A of the examination. The questions test your source comprehension skills and your ability to show your knowledge and understanding and are worth 20 marks in total.

Question 1(a) – comprehension of source material

SOURCE A

The voyages of Diaz and da Gama

What does Source A show you about the Voyages of Discovery?

[2 marks]

- *Remember to pick out at least two facts from the picture;*
- *You should also make use of the information provided in the caption;*
- *For further guidance see page 7.*

Question 1(b) – selection of knowledge and understanding of key features

Describe the methods of dealing with battle wounds during the fourteenth century.

[4 marks]

- *You must only include information that is directly relevant;*
- *You need to include a detailed and accurate description;*
- *For further guidance see page 19.*

Question 1(c) – selection of knowledge and understanding of key concepts

Look at these two sources about public health in the nineteenth century and answer the question that follows.

SOURCE B

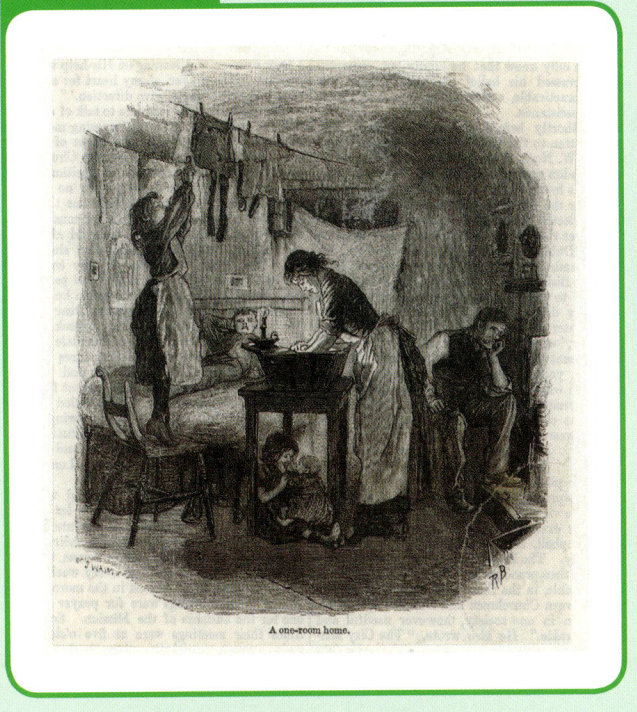

A cellar dwelling in an industrial town in the early nineteenth century

SOURCE C

In 1842 Chadwick published his findings in the *Report on the Sanitary Conditions of the Labouring Population of Great Britain...*
Chadwick recommended that local authorities should become responsible for improving drainage, removing refuse from dwellings and streets, and improving water supplies. He further recommended that a district medical officer should be appointed with responsibility for introducing sanitary improvements.

Some of Edwin Chadwick's recommendations

Use Sources B and C and your own knowledge to explain why public health improved in the nineteenth century.

[6 marks]

- *You need to use information from the sources and your own knowledge;*
- *You must refer to both sources and explain the concept of change and improvement;*
- *For further guidance see page 32.*

Question 1(d) – selection of knowledge and analysis of key concepts

How important was the work of Joseph Lister in improving patient care in the nineteenth century?

[8 marks]

- *You need to give an accurate and detailed explanation;*
- *Remember to give a reasoned judgement that targets the question;*
- *For further guidance see page 47.*

Glossary

Airman's Burn	the burns caused by burning aviation fuel when the plane's fuel tank exploded
Alchemy	a mixture of science, philosophy and magic that involved trying to change base metals into precious metals and trying to create a substance known as the philosopher's stone
Amputation	removing a part of the body, such as an arm or a leg
Arquebus	a type of muzzle-loaded gun used from the 15th to the 17th centuries
Aseptic surgery	Surgery carried out under sterile conditions
Astrology	a belief that there is a link between the movements and arrangement of the stars and people's lives
Attenuated	weaker; not as virulent
Back-to-back housing	terraced houses that share the same back wall
Base metals	metals such as iron, copper and zinc that corrode easily
Cauterise	sealing a wound with heat in order to stop it bleeding. A hot iron was used to seal blood vessels after an amputation for example, but gunshot wounds were a special case and boiling oil was used instead
Chemotherapy	the use of cell-killing drugs to treat cancer
Clinical observation	to study the condition of a patient, the treatments given and the results of the treatments
Constrained	forced
Dispensaries	a place where medicines were prepared and given out to sick people
Edema	a swelling, usually caused when fluid collects in one area of the body
Hereditary diseases	diseases that are passed on from a parent to a child
Immunosuppressive agent	a drug that stops a person's immune system rejecting a transplanted organ
Inoculation	infecting a person by injecting them with a disease to induce a milder form of it
Intravenous	injecting a substance directly into a patient's vein
Keelman	a man who worked on a special kind of flat-bottomed boat known as a keel
Keyhole surgery	operating through a very small incision, sometimes only a few centimetres long
Maternal mortality	the death of the mother during childbirth
Melancholy	a person was believed to suffer from melancholy if they were unenthusiastic and not eager for activity; today this would probably be defined as a type of depression
Miasma theory	the belief that diseases were caused by particles of decaying matter suspended in a poisonous foul smelling vapour (miasma) in the air.
Non-invasive surgery	operations performed without cutting the patient open
Pestle and mortar	the pestle is a heavy club-shaped object, which is used to crush and grind in a hard wooden, ceramic or stone bowl called a mortar
Pharmacology	a branch of science involved with studying the effects of drugs
Preventative medicine	various methods, including vaccination, of stopping people catching diseases in the first place
Puerperal fever	often called childbed fever; an infection that can be caught by women during childbirth
Purgative	a substance used to make a person vomit in order to cleanse their body

Radiotherapy	the use of radiation to treat cancer by controlling or killing malignant cells
Radiotracer	a radioactive substance that is injected into the patient so that doctors can follow its movement inside their body
Renaissance	the re-birth of old ideas in art, literature, philosophy and science, which led to new and more modern ideas
Septum	a thin membrane that divides two parts of the body, e.g. the left and right hand sides of the heart
Shrapnel	fragments of a bullet or shell
Smog	air pollution made up of smoke and fog, usually in large cities
Talisman	an object that is said to have magical powers
Tenement	a large building that housed many families. Tenements were often of a very poor quality
Vaccination	inoculating a person with a mild or inactive form of a disease in order to make them immune to that, or a different but similar, disease
Virulent	very strong, poisonous version of a disease